Know **YOUR** HCG

While most information in this book applies to all types of HCG, there can be significant differences in the following aspects:

- How to administer the HGC properly
- How to store the HCG properly

Regardless of which type of HCG is used, it is critical that YOU understand these details which are specific to the type of HCG **YOU** will be using.

Between YOU and your practitioner, complete the following:

Type of HCG:

I will be using _____ (i.e. injections, mixed sublingual, homeopathic drops, cream, etc.)

Starting Dosage Instructions of HCG:

I will be taking _____ (i.e. .5 cc, .6 cc, 1.0 cc, etc.) _____ (i.e. 1, 2, 3, etc.) times per day by _____ (i.e. under the tongue, by injection, etc.).

Additional Notes (i.e. first thing in the morning, spread out evenly, don't eat or drink for 15 minutes on either side of dose, etc):

_____

_____

_____

Proper Storage Directions:

My HCG should be stored as follows (i.e. injections - in the refrigerator, homeopathic - in a controlled environment but not necessarily refrigerated, etc.):

_____

_____

_____

It is important that YOU follow all directions carefully.

HCG Weight Loss Cure Guide

A Supplemental Guide to Dr. Simeons' Pounds and Inches Supporting All Types of HCG

A STEP BY STEP GUIDE TO MAXIMIZING YOUR HCG WEIGHT LOSS SUCCESS

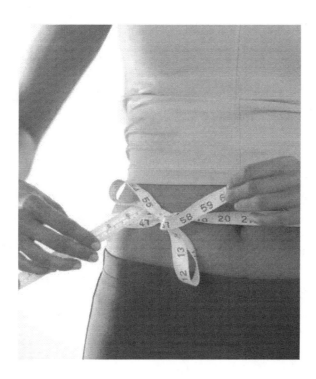

Table of Contents

Copyright Statement

Medical Disclaimer

This guide provides weight loss information and is intended only to assist users in their personal weight loss efforts. This is not written by a medical organization and offers no medical advice or diagnosis. Nothing contained in this packet should be construed as medical advice or diagnosis. The information generated should not be interpreted as a substitute for physician consultation, evaluation, or treatment.

You are urged and advised to seek the advice of a physician before beginning any weight loss effort or regimen. This information is not meant to replace the advice of any physician. Do not rely upon any information to replace consultations or advice received by qualified health professionals regarding your own specific situation. The packet is provided for your further evaluation of the information provided by Dr. A.T.W. Simeons' manuscript in *Pounds and Inches: A New Approach to Obesity* and Kevin Trudeau's book *The Weight Loss Cure They Don't Want You to Know About.* Any information included should NEVER be construed as medical advice.

If you have any question in your mind regarding any lingering health concern, you should seek medical assistance. If you are not satisfied with the advice being rendered by your current physician, you always have the right to obtain another medical opinion.

Conditions Requiring Additional Concern

If any of the following conditions apply to you, it is *strongly recommended* that you review this protocol carefully with your physician to avoid complications and/or recognize concerns. Additionally, *if you are on medications*, such as for high blood pressure and diabetes, you should be monitored by your physician because some medications require adjustment during the protocol as a natural (*and positive*) side effect of the HCG.

Gallbladder Issues – precautionary steps and additional monitoring may be warranted.
Per Dr. Simeons... Small stones in the gall bladder may in patients who have recently had typical colics cause more frequent colics under treatment with HCG...Before undertaking treatment we explain to such patients that there is a risk of more frequent and possibly severe symptoms and that it may become necessary to operate. If they are prepared to take this risk and provided they agree to undergo an operation if we consider this imperative, we proceed with treatment, as after weight reduction with HCG the operative risk is considerably reduced in an obese patient. In such cases we always give a drug which stimulates the flow of bile, and in the majority of cases nothing untoward happens. On the other hand, we have looked for and not found any evidence to suggest that the HCG treatment leads to the formation of gallstones as pregnancy sometimes does.

Gout – precautionary steps and additional monitoring may be warranted. Per Dr. Simeons... An identical behavior is found in the blood uric acid level of patients suffering from gout. Predictably such patients get an acute and often severe attack after the first few days of HCG treatment but then remain entirely free of pain, in spite of the fact that their blood uric acid often shows a marked increase which may persist for several months after treatment. Those patients who have regained their normal weight remain free of symptoms regardless of what they eat, while those that require a second course of treatment get another attack of gout as soon as the second course is initiated. We do not yet know what diencephalic mechanisms are involved in gout; possibly emotional factors play a role, and it is worth remembering that the disease does not occur in women of childbearing age. We now give 2 tablets daily of ZYLORIC to all patients who give a history of gout and have a high blood uric acid level. In this way we can completely avoid attacks during treatment.

Brittle/Unstable Diabetes – high awareness is critical.
Per Dr. Simeons ...*Diabetes* - In an obese patient suffering from a fairly advanced case of stable diabetes of many years duration in which the blood sugar may range from 300-400 mg, it is often possible to stop all anti-diabetes medication after the first few days of treatment. The blood sugar continues to drop from day to day and often reaches normal values in 2-3 weeks. As in pregnancy, this phenomenon is not observed in the brittle type of diabetes, and as some cases that are predominantly stable may have a small brittle factor in their clinical makeup, all obese diabetics have to be kept under a very careful and expert watch. A brittle case of diabetes is primarily due to the inability of the pancreas to produce sufficient insulin, while in the stable type, diencephalic regulations seem to be of greater importance. That is possibly the reason why the stable form responds so well to the HCG method of treating obesity, whereas the brittle type does not. Obese patients are generally suffering from the stable type, but a stable type may gradually change into a brittle one, which is usually associated with a loss of weight. Thus, when an obese diabetic finds that he is losing weight without diet or treatment, he should at once have his diabetes expertly attended to. There is some evidence to suggest that the change from stable to brittle is more liable to occur in patients who are taking insulin for their stable diabetes.

Fibroids – high awareness is advised. Per Dr. Simeons ...*Fibroids* - While uterine fibroids seem to be in no way affected by HCG in the doses we use, we have found that very large, externally palpable uterine myomas are apt to give trouble. We are convinced that this is entirely due to the rather sudden disappearance of fat from the pelvic bed upon which they rest and that it is the weight of the tumor pressing on the underlying tissues which accounts for the discomfort or pain which may arise during treatment. While we disregard even fair-sized or multiple myomas, we insist that very large ones be operated before treatment. We have had patients present themselves for reducing fat from their abdomen who showed no signs of obesity, but had a large abdominal tumor.

We implore anyone considering participation in any HCG protocol to read in full Dr. Simeons' *Pounds and Inches: A New Approach to Obesity*, which is in the Appendix of this book.

Regardless of whether you go to a doctor or clinic or otherwise, the manuscript provides critical background regarding HCG research and information in mostly layman terms. As with most health related issues, the final outcome or personal success depends heavily on you and your commitment to the program you choose. In other words, your success depends upon YOU! Best wishes in achieving the wonderful results that I and many others have achieved.

A Personal Opinion:

Dr. Simeons was a genius who took a couple of decades of his life to fine tune a weight loss protocol that worked quickly, was very simplistic, but had long term success. As far as I am concerned, he succeeded. Dr. Simeons wanted to provide a short term fix (unlike the diet industry and food industry) to a long term problem, and that is exactly what he did for his patients. He did not want people to need him for the rest of their lives; rather he wanted to help them fix their problem and have them move along with their lives taking very little carryover of the years spent with extra baggage, both physical and psychological, with them. The protocol parallels this goal of major short term changes (500 calorie diet) with long term results (extra weight gone) and very little carryover baggage (patients could expect to eat when they were hungry and not regain the weight back). BRAVO!

While the low calorie diet phase of the diet is limited to 500 calories per day, Dr. Simeons focused more on the simplicity of picking from the food groups, and not paying much attention to the number of calories in individual items. Other than being very specific in weighing the protein portion on one phase of the diet, his instructions appear to be intentionally vague. He even specifically indicates that the size of the apple is irrelevant; however, one may **not** substitute 2 small for one large apple.

Likewise, as you enter the maintenance phase, Dr. Simeons gets increasingly vague – again, I believe this is on purpose. In this phase, you eat as you wish with the exception of no sugars and no starches (**not** no carbohydrates), but you weigh everyday to make sure you haven't gained more than 2 pounds since your last HCG date weight. Pretty simple!

The final step is to slowly add sugars and starches. As before, you must weigh everyday to make sure you haven't gained more than 2 pounds since your last HCG date weight.

Again, in my opinion, Dr. Simeons attempts to help you get rid of your excess weight/stored fat and fix your metabolism -- possibly correcting a condition that has not worked properly your entire life. He then sends you on your way with a healthy philosophy of eating without detailed rules and regulations since a 'normal' person doesn't live by detailed rules and regulations, but rather by instinct and a healthy working body, which you should have at the successful end of his protocol!

Thank you Dr. Simeons!

Good luck and best wishes in this exciting endeavor,

Linda Prinster
Pounds and Inches Away, Inc.
www.PoundsAndInchesAway.com

Special Notes/Goals of the HCG Protocol

If you aren't familiar with all of the terms used below, do not be concerned as you will be very familiar with all of these terms once you read Dr. Simeons' manuscript (included in the Appendix of the guide) and as you go through the protocol.

There are actually three goals most people are trying to achieve by completing the HCG protocol:
   1. **Lose Weight**
   2. **Reset/Fix/Increase Base Metabolism**
   3. **Maintain Weight Loss**

Goal #1: Lose Weight, is best achieved, of course, by following the protocol 100%.

Goal #2: Reset/Fix/Improve Base Metabolism, requires the completion of a minimum 20 consecutive, non cheating, effective* HCG days on the 500 calorie diet. Performing the requirements for this goal helps with the remaining time spent on the protocol, but is even more important to your future success. It may determine whether or not you can eat good, healthy, real food like a normal, healthy person in the future. Dr. Simeons put it this way:

"We never give a treatment lasting less than 26 days, even in patients needing to lose only 5 pounds. It seems that even in the mildest cases of obesity the diencephalon requires about three weeks rest from the maximal exertion to which it has been previously subjected in order to regain fully its normal fat-banking capacity. Clinically this expresses itself, in the fact that, when in these mild cases, treatment is stopped as soon as the weight is normal, which may be achieved in a week, it is much more easily regained than after a full course of 23 injections."

"Interruptions occurring before 20 effective injections have been given are most undesirable, because with less than that number of injections some weight is liable to be regained. After the 20th injection an unavoidable interruption is merely a loss of time."

Please keep this 20, non cheating, consecutive, effective HCG days of 500 calorie diet in mind if you want to affect your metabolism both during the protocol and for the rest of your life.

*Effective HCG days do not include gorge days; only 500 calorie diet days are considered effective HCG days per Dr. Simeons' manuscript.

Goal #3: Maintain Weight Loss, is determined mainly by how well you performed the requirements for Goal #2 *(reset metabolism)* and how well you perform the maintenance phase *(also referred to as Phase 3 and P3 by Kevin Trudeau).* During the maintenance phase you try to instill a new weight set point in your body.

Besides seriously avoiding sugars and starches during the three weeks following the HCG phase, even if you don't go over your maintenance weight, you should attempt to keep your weight as steady as possible during this phase to reach a new weight set point in your body. It seems the faster this is done and the more consistent one stays at a weight, the quicker the body takes over in making sure the new weight is maintained (instead of us watching so closely and 'manipulating' weight changes by eating carefully or doing Steak Days), without stressing us out. This is when we want our bodies to take on the new weight set point.

Avoiding sugars and starches also helps us achieve the goal of maintaining weight loss because most people crave less and are satisfied with less than they used to be when they do choose to indulge.

Please be aware of all three goals and what each requires as you execute the different phases of the protocol in order to achieve ultimate, long-term success.

Summary of a Typical Round

Day 1 and 2: Take HCG and gorge. Dr. Simeons emphasized that these days should be spent eating as much fattening food as possible to restore structural fat and avoid hunger at start up.

Starting with Day 3: Take HCG and follow 500 calorie diet plan for up to 40 days (except during menstruation – during menstruation Dr. Simeons advised to not take HCG, but to continue the 500 calorie diet -- some participants stop the HCG for the whole time; some stop HCG during heavy days only; some never stop, but continue HCG straight through menstruation).

Sometime after 23 HCG days, but before 41 HCG days: Stop HCG, continue following the 500 calorie diet for 72 hours/3days after last HCG.

Note: Dr. Simeons manuscript (included in the Appendix of this book) mentions staying on the 500 calorie diet for '3 days' a couple of places and '72 hours' at least one place. While these appear to be the same, if you are taking HCG in the morning, these terms would make the difference of a day.

For example, let us say that you take your last dose of HCG on Monday morning at 8:00 a.m. If you follow the '3 day' verbiage, then you would count your non HCG days as Tuesday, Wednesday and Thursday. Under this scenario, you would begin the maintenance phase eating on Friday morning.

On the other hand, if you follow the '72 hour' verbiage, then you would count your 72 hours as follows: from Monday at 8:00 a.m. to Tuesday at 8:00 a.m. is 24 hours, Tuesday to Wednesday at 8:00 a.m. is 48 hours, and Wednesday to Thursday at 8:00 a.m. is 72 hours. Under this scenario, you would begin the maintenance phase eating on Thursday at 8:00 a.m.

At this point in your protocol, either interpretation is probably acceptable. We actually recommend using the 3rd full day as a transition day when you have 2 eggs for breakfast and spend the rest of the day eating the same 500 calorie diet.

Another way to decide how to handle the 3rd day is by following your appetite. If you are starving on the 3rd full day, the HCG is probably out of your system, so maintenance is appropriate. On the other hand, if you are not hungry, there is probably still some HCG in your system and the 500 calorie diet is still appropriate. If you aren't feeling either starving or full, then a transition day is safe both psychologically and physically.

Maintenance: refer to "What can I eat and drink" section of this manual for helpful information about what you can and cannot eat/drink during all phases of the diet.

1st 3 weeks after stopping HCG: All foods are allowed except starches and sugars, always controlled by morning weighing*.

2nd 3 weeks after stopping HCG: Very gradually add starches and sugars in small quantities, always controlled by morning weighing*.

The future: Continue controlling by morning weighing.*

*Weigh daily and execute a Steak Day** on any morning that your weight is more than 2 pounds over your weight as of last HCG dose.

**Steak Day: "Skip breakfast and lunch but take plenty to drink. In the evening, eat a huge steak with only an apple or a raw tomato." Dr. Simeons

Getting Started

1) Read in full Dr. Simeons' *Pounds and Inches: A New Approach to Obesity,* which is in the Appendix of this book. Otherwise, you will not have a comfortable knowledge and feeling with this protocol and you may not be familiar with many terms in this guide.

2) You should check with your physician before beginning any weight loss program.

3) If you may be combining HCG with other medications, you should discuss this with your physician and you may also want to do some research on your own using drug interaction tools such as http://www.medscape.com/druginfo/druginterchecker?src=google.

4) Once you have decided to proceed with Dr. Simeons' HCG protocol, acquire the HCG and HCG supplies (see HCG 'Types' on page 10), a quality digital bathroom scale that measures in increments of .1 or .2 pounds (tenths) and a quality food scale that measures in grams. A George Forman grill (or similar) is also a very good investment.

5) (Optional)If you have some time before you obtain your HCG or cannot start for a couple of weeks for some other reason, your time might be well spent by completing a Candida colon cleanse and/or a gall bladder cleanse. These can be found at your neighborhood health store or online. Any cleanse doesn't need to be drastic or cause you to suffer since it is just a primer for your upcoming weight loss protocol and it may reduce cravings as you begin the protocol.

6) Pick your starting date. If you are a menstruating woman, refer to Dr. Simeons' manuscript regarding what time to avoid starting the protocol.

7) Take 'Before' pictures from front, side and back profile. Also, take measurements and record them on the 'Tracking Your Progress' form in this guide. Determine your goal weight based on input from your physician and the appropriate weight chart included in this guide.

8) If you are using an HCG type that requires mixing, such as Injection HCG or Mixed, Sublingual HCG (Homeopathic HCG does not require mixing), decide your starting dose. The day before you intend to start the two day gorge, prepare your solution and store the mixed HCG in the refrigerator. Refrigeration is required for Injection HCG and Mixed, Sublingual HCG (Homeopathic HCG does not require refrigeration).

9) On your starting date, which **is** your first gorge day, begin taking HCG on a consistent schedule. (See directions for your specific type of HCG.)

10) The first two HCG days are your 'load' or 'gorge' days. Dr. Simeons emphasized that these days should be spent eating as much fattening food as possible to restore structural fat and avoid hunger at startup. (See Sample Gorge Days on page 28.)

11) Starting with the 3rd HCG day, use the 500 Calorie Diet and continue until 72 hours after the last HCG day. Try to eat 'real', natural food (avoiding antibiotics, chemical/sugared injections, and frozen glazes with ingredients you can't pronounce).

What to expect during the 1st week…

- Possibly a headache as you detox from sodas, sugar, etc. (aspirin is allowed)
- Some hunger or minor discomfort , if you don't gorge sufficiently, usually peaking around the 5th day of the protocol
- An overall feeling of well-being; sometimes quite a euphoric feeling with lots of energy
- Fluctuations in weight loss – "After the fourth or fifth day of dieting the daily loss of weight begins to decrease to one pound or somewhat less per day…Men often continue to lose regularly at that rate, but women are more irregular in spite of faultless dieting. There may be no drop at all for two or three days and then a sudden loss which reestablishes the normal average. These fluctuations are entirely due to variations in the retention and elimination of water, which are more marked in women than in men." Dr. Simeons
- Blood Sugar – "Towards the end of a course or when a patient has nearly reached his normal weight it occasionally happens that the blood sugar drops below normal... Such an attack of hypoglycemia … comes on suddenly; there is the same feeling of light-headedness, weakness in the knees, trembling, and unmotivated sweating. But under HCG, hypoglycemia does not produce any feeling of hunger. All these symptoms are almost instantly relieved by taking two heaped teaspoons of sugar." Dr. Simeons

12) Per the manuscript the minimum number of HCG days for a cycle is 23 with a maximum per cycle of 40 HCG days. Note: You continue the 500 Calorie Diet for three days after the last dose of HCG. *There are a few exceptions that should be reviewed in the manuscript such as what to do if you reach your goal weight before completing 23 HCG days. (See Duration of Treatment in the manuscript located in the appendix of this guide).

13) The first 3 weeks after stopping HCG, all foods are allowed except starches and sugars (must use caution with very sweet fruit such as melons, grapes, bananas). See tips on this 'maintenance phase' also known as Phase 3 or P3 as it is referred to in Kevin Trudeau's *The Weight Loss Cure They Don't Want You to Know About*. Weigh daily and execute a steak day on any morning that your weight is more than 2 pounds over your weight as of last HCG dose.

14) After next 3 weeks after stopping HCG (weeks 4-6 after stopping HCG), very gradually add sugar and starch in small quantities. As in the above 3 weeks, weigh daily and execute a steak day on any morning that your weight is more than 2 pounds over your weight as of last HCG dose.

15) If you have reached your goal, congratulations and enjoy your new body! If you choose to lose more weight with additional rounds, continue to take the above 6 week break at a minimum per Dr. Simeons' strong recommendation -- more time is suggested between round 2 and round 3, etc.

Beware of the Following Roadblocks
… These can stop you dead in your tracks!

Spices – All ingredients (not just the nutritional information) must be analyzed to ensure no sugar, starch, oil, fats or other unallowable items are included. Read more about spices on the next page. Be aware that even Stevia products often have some form of sugar added to improve taste. Therefore, some brands of Stevia should not be used during the low calorie phase i.e. Truvia and several others.

HRT (Hormone Replacement Therapy) – While the thought of stopping successful HRT may be terrifying; participating in the HCG protocol with little to no weight loss is even more terrifying. The good news is that participants report that HCG keeps many of the symptoms HRT is being used for at bay, so weight loss can be achieved while taking a short leave from HRT without undue hardship. This must be carefully considered and should be undertaken with your physician. Theoretically, the participant knows what symptoms to watch for, and can go back to HRT (if required) on short notice.

Some Medicines i.e. Steroids – Most prescription medicines do NOT seem to have an adverse affect on the protocol such as high blood pressure, cholesterol, etc. However, some, such as steroids, do. If weight gain is a common side effect of a given medication, this should raise a red flag. Any medications taken in an oily substance (ear drops; ointments) are also suspect. Any change in medication should not be taken without serious consideration and consultation with your physician.

Beef – Extra caution is needed due to the high fat content in American beef. It is advisable to not have ground beef or roast more than 2-3 times per week (or none is fine, also). Lean steaks such as sirloin and filet usually have better results.

Best Advice…Be Intentional…A Philosophy of Sorts

When beginning an HCG diet protocol, we find it imperative to impress upon clients the requirement to *BE INTENTIONAL.* This applies to everything you eat and everything that comes in contact with your skin.

While we follow Dr. Simeons' protocol, there are other HCG protocols that differ —some to a slight degree and others to a large degree. Dr. Simeons worked on his protocol for about 20 years, and we feel confident that he knew EXACTLY what he was talking about. So, for example, when someone says, "Well, green beans and broccoli are really good for you AND every other diet lets you have those, so why can't we have those?" or "Do you really think they will hurt anything?" OR, my personal all-time favorite, "I ate them and they didn't make any difference!"…Our response is "I guarantee you that Dr. Simeons didn't just forget about green beans and broccoli, only to remember beet greens and fennel. I guarantee he tried them, and that the results were simply not as favorable." In summary, no one knows for sure that bending the rules did NOT 'hurt' them. For example, if they mixed vegetables or ate un-allowed vegetables, or did other slight variances, a person doesn't know how much they would have lost if they had NOT mixed vegetables or NOT had green beans or NOT had a seasoning spice that contained sugar or starch in some, small form.

We have seen many people stall due to seasonings. You must realize that something as harmless as garlic salt may have several ingredients that potentially stall you -- even just a few sprinkles. It is a common occurrence for us to have clients get all of their spices out at one time and read us all ingredients – not the food nutritional values; but the actual ingredients. When one person stalled she reported only using salt, pepper, and garlic salt. The problem was that the 'innocent' garlic salt had both sugar and modified corn starch listed as ingredients. If you think this can't stall you, we have found differently. So, with regard to spices – BE INTENTIONAL.

If your hands or lips are dry, you might try to get by without your typical hand lotion or Burt's Bees Wax. And then you might try to get by with just mineral oil; however, at some point before you actually bleed, you may have to put a slight amount of healing lotion on your hands twice a day or sparsely apply medicated Blistex to your lips just twice a day– BE INTENTIONAL.

If your George Foreman grill is starting to stick to food, you may decide to spray the grill with nonstick cooking spray. Be aware that ¼ of a second is a 'serving' and that it doesn't take many sprays to add some nutritional value to your food. So, BE INTENTIONAL and spray very quickly.

One client had an ear blockage for which her doctor prescribed an oil based ear drop. With just a few drops, she gained 3 pounds – we know it doesn't make sense with our common knowledge, but it also doesn't matter that it doesn't make sense. Since her condition had been building for some time and didn't require immediate treatment, she stopped the oil until she was done with her current HCG cycle – BE INTENTIONAL. (P.S. She did proceed with her treatment after the cycle and, of course, did not gain weight because the HCG was then out of her system.)

You will find several people who boast about losing weight while cheating, mixing vegetables, using un-allowed spices, having salsa, drinking alcohol here and there, etc. While they have continued to lose, please always remember that it only means that they could have possibly lost more AND that they may be bypassing the opportunity for resetting their metabolism to the fullest extent possible, thereby jeopardizing their future weight maintenance capabilities. So, minimize stretching or compromising any rules, in any way, for medical, social or other reasons—ALWAYS BE INTENTIONAL in order to maximize the overall effect on your incredible weight loss journey.

About HCG

Q. What is HCG?

A. HCG (Human Chorionic Gonadotropin) is a hormone naturally produced in large quantity during pregnancy. Dr. ATW Simeons, the doctor who developed and worked with the protocol for about 20 years, found that small regular doses of HCG caused the body to release abnormal fat when used in conjunction with a specific 500 calorie daily diet. This is detailed in Dr. Simeons' manuscript ***Pounds and Inches: A New Approach to Obesity,*** which is in the appendix of this book. For a full description of what HCG is and why Dr. Simeons proposes that HCG makes weight loss and maintenance at a new weight level possible, you simply must read Dr. Simeons full manuscript which is included in the appendix of this guide.

HCG 'Types'

Until recently, most participants relied on HCG injections as the only consistent, effective method of using HCG for weight loss. However, support of additional HCG types including two different types of sublingual (under the tongue) HCG and prescription HCG cream have become more popular as experience and some results remain comparable to HCG injections. While most information in this book applies to all types of HCG, there can be significant differences in the following aspects:

- How to administer the HGC properly
- How to store the HCG properly

Regardless of which type of HCG is used, it is critical that each participant understands these details which are specific to the type of HCG chosen.

To be clear, there are 3 types, or methods, of HCG detailed in this book:

Type 1: Homeopathic HCG; Professional strength, homeopathic, HCG, which is made in a U.S. laboratory and does not require mixing, to be taken sublingually (under the tongue) - referred to as *Homeopathic HCG* throughout this guide.

Type 2: HCG Injections; HCG ampoule (i.e. Pregnyl, Organon) mixed with bacteriostatic water in a sterile environment to be taken by injection--referred to as *HCG Injections* throughout this guide.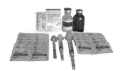

Type 3: Mixed, Sublingual HCG; HCG ampoule (i.e. Pregnyl, Organon) mixed with vitamin B12 or similar to be taken sublingually (under the tongue)--referred to as *Mixed, Sublingual HCG* throughout this guide.

Again, if you are using another type of HCG i.e. cream, spray, etc, make sure you understand the proper use and storage, and follow all directions carefully.

The features of each of the three HCG Types are listed below.

	Type 1: Homeopathic HCG (Taken sublingually) A professional strength homeopathic made in a U.S. lab; no mixing required	Type 2: Injection HCG (Prescription HCG mixed by you or pharmacist)	Type 3: Sublingual, Mixed HCG (Prescription HCG mixed with B12 or other by you or pharmacist)
Pain	None	Little to None	None
Taste	Almost tasteless	None	Depends on mixing solution i.e. B12 tastes like the liquid baby vitamins used in the 1970s
Time	4 minutes if you take it 2x per day; 6 minutes if you take it 3x per day	About 1 minute; once per day	2 minutes; twice per day
Fear	None	Usually none after 1st time, but can be high anxiety before	None
Average Weight Loss per Cycle	With committed participants, 20 – 30 lbs. in 30 – 40 diet days	With committed participants, 20 – 30 lbs. in 30 – 40 diet days	With committed participants, 20 – 30 lbs. in 30 – 40 diet days

We have experience with all three types of HCG listed above and know that, if used correctly with quality HCG, all three methods are very effective.

Sites and Forums Supporting HCG Protocols

If you need further information or would like to ask other participants questions to help you further in deciding which type of HCG to use, the following web sites are all up and running as of July, 2009. These can be a great resource when you need moral support, questions answered, and extra confidence in what you are doing. Most of these do not claim medical advice, but are built around participants like you. Some nurses and doctors participate in some forums just like you and me, so the HCG protocol has a great deal of interest right now. Without the complete medical support offered in Dr. Simeons' clinic (daily meeting with each patient), these forums are places you can go to ask if others are on the same medications as you, or any other circumstances, just to get a feel for what others, like you, are doing and experiencing. None of this information is a substitute for your medical physician in any way, shape or form and should not be construed as such. This is unqualified information that many find extremely valuable, encouraging and motivating. Only you can judge if any of this information is of any value to YOU.

Some of these sites require you to request membership. From what I gather, this is to keep the 'HCG bashers' off the site, but again, you be the judge.

> http://www.HCGdietinfo.com/
> http://health.groups.yahoo.com/group/HCGDIET/
> http://HCGsupportgroup.forumotion.com/

Other HCG sites you may find helpful from http://health.groups.yahoo.com/group/HCGDIET/ :
> FAQ:http://www.HCGdietinfo.com/HCG-Weight-Loss-FAQ.htm
> Personal Care Products: http://www.HCGdietinfo.com/HCG-Diet-Products.htm

Type 1: Homeopathic HCG Specific Use Instructions

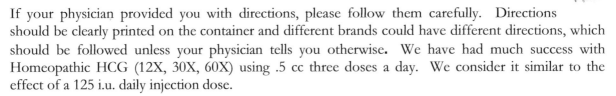

Administering Homeopathic HCG - Sublingual Use ONLY

If your physician provided you with directions, please follow them carefully. Directions should be clearly printed on the container and different brands could have different directions, which should be followed unless your physician tells you otherwise. We have had much success with Homeopathic HCG (12X, 30X, 60X) using .5 cc three doses a day. We consider it similar to the effect of a 125 i.u. daily injection dose.

Daily Instructions: 3 Times per Day, shake the HCG solution each time before drawing the Homeopathic HCG solution into the dropper or oral syringe. Deposit .5cc (the same as ½ cc or ½ ml) of Homeopathic HCG under your tongue and let it sit there for 2 minutes before swallowing. Both before and after taking the HCG, avoid eating, drinking and/or smoking for 15 minutes to allow the most effective absorption.

Special Condition: If someone has a particularly strenuous or inconsistent life schedule i.e. odd work shifts or no long period of sleep per day, some participants reported more consistent results by taking the HCG four times per day, evenly spread out through awake time.

For information on adjusting the dose with Homeopathic HCG Dose refer to Page 19.

Proper Storage of Homeopathic HCG

For Homeopathic HCG, the sealed bottles can be stored at room temperature until you are ready to use it. Once Homeopathic HCG is opened, the HCG does not require refrigeration to last for a complete round. However, the HCG should not be subject to extreme temperature changes. For example, keeping the HCG in your car may not be a good idea due to local climate, but keeping the HCG in your purse is usually fine since it stays with you, and therefore stays at a reasonable temperature.

Additionally, if you have some Homeopathic HCG leftover at the end of a cycle that you would like to use to begin another round in 6 weeks or soon after, your HCG should be stored in the refrigerator during the break for better preservation. Depending on temperature variances, microwave exposure, and other circumstances, the leftover HCG may or may not be good for a couple of months.

If you start to feel extremely bad, the potency of your HCG could be the culprit. You would also evaluate if you have potentially achieved your ideal weight or if immunity may be an issue. Dr. Simeons manuscript covers this well, so be on the lookout if you ever start feeling unusually drained – an extremely wiped out feeling.

Additional Homeopathic HCG Directions

- Do NOT store by microware, in direct sunlight or near x-ray.
- Take nothing by mouth 15 minutes prior to or following dosage. This includes food, drink, cigarettes, chewing gum, toothpaste, any mint (i.e. candy, mouthwash) or camphor products etc.
- Avoid camphor, as in muscle and joint rubs, and moth balls fumes.
- If dental trauma to mouth occurs, use only topically for 48 hours i.e. if you have dental drilling in the back your mouth, apply the HCG on the outside of your gums on the front left side.
- Limit breathing of strong smells, i.e.as paint thinner, cigarette smoke for one hour after dose.
- Limit raw garlic, onions and strong spices to one hour after taking HCG.
- Do not want to expose the bottle to extreme high or low temperatures.

Type 2: HCG Injection Specific Use Instructions

Administering HCG Injections

Helpful Notes Regarding HCG Diet Shots

1 ml = 1 cc

If you do not know how to administer shots, consult with your physician or some other qualified person to either teach you how to properly self-inject OR simply have a qualified person give you the shots. Millions of diabetics and others give themselves shots on a daily basis. Participants usually have more of a mental block regarding self-injection than a physical issue. Most participants are very comfortable self-injecting within the first week. However, most participants do know someone who is qualified to give injections because of past or personal experience, and this helps the more hesitant participants get comfortable with the injection until self-injection is possible. Below are some helpful tips in the process of self-injecting HCG.

This does not replace your physician's advice or constitute medical advice, but only tips of the trade.

Loading a Syringe in Preparation for Injection

1. Clean the exposed rubber seal of your sealed vial using an alcohol swab.
2. Remove the syringe from the plastic or paper cover—this should be as easy as pulling two pieces of plastic away from each other when done correctly. If needles and syringes are in two pieces, attach the needle securely. If the needles are not insulin needles, but are already together when you receive them, tighten the needle on the syringe to avoid leakage, as they can shake slightly loose during shipping.
3. With the needle capped, pull back the plunger, which will fill the syringe with air equal to the amount of HCG solution to be drawn, i.e. pull back to ½ cc if drawing up ½ cc of HCG solution.
4. Remove the cap covering the needle and set it on its side to prevent contamination. Be careful not to touch the needle. The inside of the cap and needle is sterile, and the needle will be covered again with this cap.
5. With the vial in an up-right position, push the needle through the cleansed rubber stopper on the vial. Push the needle in at a 90 degree angle, being careful not to bend the needle.
6. Inject the air in the syringe into the vial.
7. Turn the vial upside down, with the needle remaining in the vial. The needle will be pointing upward. Make sure that the tip of the needle is completely covered by the medication. This will make it easier to withdraw the solution (and not air).
8. Pull back on the plunger to fill the syringe with the correct dose of solution. Keep the vial upside down, with the needle in the vial pointed upward until there are no big air bubbles. If you have air bubbles, tap the syringe, or "flick" it with your fingertips. Once the bubbles are at the top of the syringe, gently push on the plunger to force the bubbles out of the syringe and back into the vial. Note: It is important to eliminate large air bubbles because they take up space needed for the medication.
9. Turn the vial and needle upright, being careful not to bend the needle.
10. Pull the needle straight out and recap if you are not administering the injection immediately, i.e. if you fill 7 syringes at a time, carefully replace the needle cap to prevent contamination and store loaded syringes in a closed sterile container in the refrigerator until ready to use.

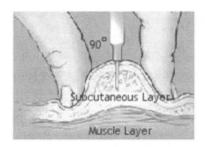

Hints on How to Administer HCG Injections
Common Subcutaneous Injection Sites

1. Clean the area with an alcohol swab in a circular motion, from center out.

2. Allow the alcohol to air dry completely to avoid stinging with the shot.

3. For intramuscular injections, gently pinch the skin and insert the needle directly into the muscle at one of the designated areas i.e. upper back hip with medical assistance or leg (check with your physician). If you are not using an insulin needle, but are instead using a 25 – 27 gauge needle/syringe combination (consult with your physician or some other qualified person to teach you how to properly self-inject is highly recommended), pull back on the syringe plunger slightly to check for blood in the syringe. If blood comes back in the syringe, the entire needle should be discarded and the process started over with a new syringe.

4. For subcutaneous injections, gently pinch the skin and insert the needle into the area between the skin and muscle at one of the designated subcutaneous areas i.e. arm, abdomen, or leg. If you are not using an insulin needle, but are instead using a 25 – 27 gauge needle/syringe combination, pull back on the syringe plunger slightly to check for blood in the syringe. If blood comes back in the syringe, the entire needle should be discarded and the process started over with a new syringe.

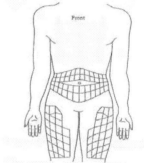

5. If the skin is still pinched, release the pinch.

6. Inject the contents of the syringe at a quick and steady pace.

Common Injection Sites

Note: It is not abnormal to see a small amount of bleeding at the injection site after the needle is removed. Direct pressure will stop the bleeding and prevent bruising of the skin. Slight swelling, redness, burning, or itching is not uncommon and should subside shortly.

Other tips to ease any discomfort associated with injections.

✓ Try a quick motion shot where you put the needle in like a dart with one fast motion vs. resting the needle on the pinched skin and pushing it through in a smooth motion to see which is more comfortable for you.

✓ Try to relax prior to injection.

✓ Apply ice to numb the location prior to injection.

✓ Rotate injection sites.

✓ Allow medications that have been refrigerated to warm to room temperature before injection.

For information on adjusting the dose with HCG Injections refer to on page 19.

Proper Storage of HCG Injections

For HCG Injections, prior to mixing, the HCG should be kept in a dark box at room temperature until the HCG is needed. HCG should be used before the expiration date, which is generally printed on the box. Several companies report expiration dates about three years from current date. **Once these types of HCG are mixed, the HCG must be stored in the refrigerator and should be potent for at least 30 days** although some brands will claim slightly longer potency.

If you start to feel extremely bad, the potency of your HCG could be the culprit. You would also evaluate if you have potentially achieved your ideal weight or if immunity may be an issue. Dr. Simeons manuscript covers this well, so be on the lookout if you ever start feeling unusually drained – an extremely wiped out feeling.

Warning: While some participants in the past have been advised to freeze HCG until you are ready to use it, this is generally not accepted as proper storage and may affect potency. Therefore, this is not recommended.

Proper Storage and Disposal of Used Needles and Syringes

Needles should be disposed of in a safe manner. Puncture resistant containers made specifically for needle disposal are called Sharps. Sharps can be purchased online, through medical supply stores, and in some pharmacies. However, there is a no cost alternative that may vary based on where you live. For example, as of September 2007, per St. Charles County Environmental Services in St. Charles County, Missouri, the following procedure is environmentally compliant:

1.) Avoid Recapping needle.
2.) Place in a heavy-duty puncture resistant container: empty liquid detergent or bleach bottle
3.) Add one teaspoon of bleach
4.) Secure lid with duct tape; write "MEDICAL WASTE" in permanent ink.
5.) Dispose in trash – NOT with recyclables

Never use coffee cans, milk jugs or glass containers for needle disposal!

Type 3: Mixed, Sublingual HCG Specific Use Instructions

Administering Mixed, Sublingual HCG – For Sublingual Use ONLY

If your physician provided you with directions, please follow them carefully. If your HCG was mixed using the instructions in this guide, the following directions have worked well for many participants.

Daily Instructions: 2 Times Per Day, Gently mix the HCG solution each time before drawing the Mixed, Sublingual HCG solution into the oral syringe. Using the oral syringe, deposit .5cc (the same as ½ cc or ½ ml) of Mixed, Sublingual HCG under your tongue and let it sit there for 2 minutes before swallowing. Both before and after taking the HCG, avoid eating, drinking and/or smoking for 15 minutes to allow the most effective absorption.

Note: the common consensus is to take a 125 i.u. dose in the morning and again in the late afternoon/early evening. Since absorption is a factor, this is thought to have the effect of a 150 i.u. - 200 i.u. daily injection dose.

For information on adjusting the dose with Mixed, Sublingual HCG Dose refer to Page 19.

Proper Storage of Mixed, Sublingual HCG

For Mixed, Sublingual HCG, prior to mixing, the HCG should be kept in a dark box at room temperature until the HCG is needed. HCG should be used before the expiration date, which is generally printed on the box. Several companies report expiration dates about three years from current date. **Once these types of HCG are mixed, the HCG must be stored in the refrigerator and should be potent for at least 30 days** although some brands will claim slightly longer potency.

If you start to feel extremely bad, the potency of your HCG could be the culprit. You would also evaluate if you have potentially achieved your ideal weight or if immunity may be an issue. Dr. Simeons manuscript covers this well, so be on the lookout if you ever start feeling unusually drained – an extremely wiped out feeling.

HCG Servicers

Pounds and Inches Away Inc., was founded in 2007 by Linda Prinster, the author of this book, The HCG Weight Loss Cure Guide. The company has supported over 1000 successful clients with the HCG Diet Protocol and much of this book has been fined tuned based on those great, detailed experiences. Check www.PoundsAndInchesAway.com for before and after pictures, videos, and testimonials if you have any doubt about whether the HCG protocol, as written by Dr. Simeons in Pounds and Inches: A New Approach to Obesity, is everything it is touted to be.

In other words, the HCG protocol works. Unless a required medication is interfering, almost 100% of participants SHOULD be successful in losing over 20 pounds (if a participant has this much to lose) in a 40 day cycle if the protocol is followed correctly. If a participant is not having success and medications are not the problem, experienced support should be able to make the difference between expected results (over 20 pounds in a cycle) and less effective or no results.

For support options, search on the web or inquire on the various HCG forums for a provider with whom you are comfortable and confident Since the first publication of this guide, there are many more practitioners, both medical and nonmedical, offering support for the HCG Diet Protocol. Be aware that different providers vary significantly in cost, support, and knowledge. Therefore, it is important to ask questions and get personal referrals, if possible, before choosing a provider.

Adjustments to HCG Dosage during a Cycle

There are many physicians, clinics, and individuals using many different strengths of HCG at this time. Dr. Simeons only used injections, no sublingual, and generally started everyone on 125 i.u. dose per daily injection. Under certain circumstances, some listed below; the daily dosage is increased, as necessary, in small increments.

Many participants increase the daily injection dosage strength by about 25 i.u. at a time (waiting a day or two in between adjustments) for one or more of the following reasons:
  ➤ the participant continues to be very hungry after the first week when hunger should be less
  ➤ energy continues to be quite low
  ➤ slowed weight loss
  ➤ slight signs of immunity
  ➤ potency concerns (HCG has been mixed and refrigerated for close to a month)

To increase the HCG dose during a round, increase the amount of HCG drawn into the syringe (for either injection, mixed sublingual or homeopathic) for each dose as follows without needing to re-mix or potentially waste any HCG:

Amount to draw into syringe	=	Correlating Dosage in international units
Approximately .5 cc	=	125 i.u. (approximately 40 days) Dr. Simeons' starting dose
Approximately .6 cc	=	150 i.u. (approximately 33 days)
Approximately .7 cc	=	175 i.u. (approximately 28 days)
Approximately .8 cc	=	200 i.u. (approximately 25 days)

For Homeopathic HCG, our experience has led us to start with .5 cc three times per day. If the above conditions exist, participants increase by .1 cc three times per day, i.e. from .5 cc to .6 cc three times per day (waiting a day or two in between adjustments to see if the conditions subside or improve).

For Injection HCG, our experience has led us to start with .5 cc one time per day. If the above conditions exist, participants increase by .1 cc one time per day, i.e. from .5 cc to .6 cc one time per day (waiting a day or two in between adjustments to see if the conditions subside or improve).

For Mixed, Sublingual HCG, our experience has led us to start with .5 cc twice a day. Rarely, if the above conditions exist, participants increase by .1 cc two times per day, i.e. from .5 cc to .6 cc two times per day (waiting a day or two in between adjustments to see if the conditions subside or improve).

Preparation Phase (Phase 1 as referenced in Trudeau's book)

Phase 1, as referenced in Kevin Trudeau's book, is an optional phase added to the front of Dr. Simeons' HCG protocol. This added phase is not required for successful weight loss although there may be health benefits from some of the suggestions, such as completing a good Candida colon cleanse, etc.

Kevin Trudeau's book, _The Weight Loss Cure They Don't Want You to Know About,_ goes much further into health issues than Dr. Simeons' protocol, which was focused more narrowly on losing abnormal fat/weight. For example, Trudeau's book suggests eating 100% organic, getting many colonics, drinking many exotic teas, and many, many other health-oriented suggestions. While we believe some of these suggestions are healthy alternatives and good ideas, these suggestions are not required for successful weight loss using Dr. Simeons' original HCG protocol. Also, we consider some of these ideas easier to implement or 'work toward' after losing the weight instead of trying to implement too many drastic changes at one time into our already busy lives.

Therefore, we actually recommend reading Kevin Trudeau's book after successfully losing your weight using Dr. Simeons' protocol (in the appendix of this book). Otherwise, Trudeau's book tends to give the impression that losing the weight is an expensive, complicated process when it simply does not have to be.

If you do have a couple of weeks before you start the HCG protocol, many participants have suggested that a good colon cleanse or some other systematic cleanses can help you feel better and cut down on the cravings during the diet phase. Many participants also lose a few pounds if they do a cleanse or two. So, this can get you moving in the right direction and build momentum as you get ready to start the protocol and gather your HCG and other protocol supplies.

Since gallbladder issues can be complicated or aggravated by the HCG protocol or losing significant weight with any plan, you may also consider doing a gallbladder/liver cleanse either before or immediately after completing the very low calorie phase of the diet. Gallbladder issues seem to occur quite soon after moving into maintenance, so the sooner the better if you are considering this type of cleanse, especially if you know you have a history of gallbladder issues.

As you prepare to participate in the 500 calorie/Very Low Calorie Diet Phase of the HCG protocol, keep the following ultimate goal in mind: To Live a healthy life without constantly fighting your own body on food/weight issues.

If you think completing the HCG protocol is difficult, try reminding yourself that you can do anything for a month (about one cycle) and worry about the rest (if you need more than one cycle) when the time comes, from a new and improved place in your life (as you will probably be down 20-30 pounds at that time).

500 Calorie Diet (P2 or Phase 2 as referenced in Trudeau's book)

(Below is from Simeons except words in parenthesis () have been added for clarification purposes.)

The Diet

The 500 calorie diet is explained on the day of the second injection to those patients who will be preparing their own food, and it is most important that the person who will actually cook is present - the wife, the mother or the cook, as the case may be. Here in Italy patients are given the following diet sheet.

Breakfast:	Tea or coffee in any quantity without sugar. Only one tablespoonful of milk allowed in 24 hours. Saccharin or Stevia may be used.
Lunch:	1. 100 grams of veal, beef, chicken breast, fresh white fish, lobster, crab, or shrimp. All visible fat must be carefully removed before cooking, and the meat must be weighed raw. It must be boiled or grilled without additional fat. Salmon, eel, tuna, herring, dried or pickled fish are **not** allowed. The chicken breast must be removed from the bird. 2. One type of vegetable only to be chosen from the following: spinach, chard, chicory, beet-greens, green salad, tomatoes, celery, fennel, onions, red radishes, cucumbers, asparagus, cabbage. 3. One breadstick (grissino) or one Melba toast. 4. An apple or a handful of strawberries or one-half grapefruit, orange* (*in the original manuscript, but not in at least one version of the circulating manuscripts)
Dinner :	The same four choices as lunch.

The juice of one lemon daily is allowed for all purposes. Salt, pepper, vinegar, mustard powder, garlic, sweet basil, parsley, thyme, marjoram, etc., may be used for seasoning, but no oil, butter or dressing.

Tea, coffee, plain water, or mineral water are the only drinks allowed, but they may be taken in any quantity and at all times. (Green teas and plain herbal teas are USUALLY o.k., but if they list any fruit i.e. White Peach Tea or Raspberry Tea, then the tea should be avoided. Check ingredients for any fruits, vegetables, and/or oils. It is not uncommon to see orange or lemon peel, strawberry extract, carrots, peppermint oil, etc. in tea bags. The ingredients, not just the nutritional facts, must be checked thoroughly.)

In fact, the patient should drink about 2 liters of these fluids per day. Many patients are afraid to drink so much because they fear that this may make them retain more water. This is a wrong notion as the body is more inclined to store water when the intake falls below its normal requirements.

The fruit or the breadstick may be eaten between meals instead of with lunch or dinner, but not more than four items listed for lunch and dinner may be eaten at one meal.

No medicines or cosmetics other than lipstick, eyebrow pencil and powder may he used without special permission. **(NOTE: Do NOT change or discontinue prescribed medications without discussion with your physician.)**

Every item in the list is gone over carefully, continually stressing the point that no variations other than those listed may be introduced. All things not listed are forbidden, and the patient is assured that nothing permissible has been left out. The 100 grams of meat must he scrupulously weighed raw after all visible fat has been removed. To do this accurately the patient must have a letter-scale, as kitchen scales are not sufficiently accurate and the butcher should certainly not be relied upon. Those not uncommon patients, who feel that even so little food is too much for them, can omit anything they wish.

There is no objection to breaking up the two meals, for instance, having a breadstick and an apple for breakfast or before going to bed, provided they are deducted from the regular meals. The whole daily ration of two breadsticks or two fruits may not be eaten at the same time, nor can any item saved from the previous day be added on the following day. In the beginning, patients are advised to check every meal against their diet sheet before starting to eat and not to rely on their memory. It is also worth pointing out that any attempt to observe this diet without HCG will lead to trouble in two to three days. We have had cases in which patients have proudly flaunted their dieting powers in front of their friends without mentioning the fact that they are also receiving treatment with HCG. They let their friends try the same diet, and when this proves to be a failure - as it necessarily must - the patient starts raking in unmerited kudos for superhuman willpower.

It should also be mentioned that two small apples, weighing as much as one large one, never the less, have a higher caloric value and are, therefore, not allowed though there is no restriction on the size of one apple.

Some people do not realize that chicken breast does not mean the breast of any other fowl, nor does it mean a wing or drumstick.

The most tiresome patients are those who start counting calories and then come up with all manner of ingenious variations which they compile from their little books. When one has spent years of weary research trying to make a diet as attractive as possible without jeopardizing the loss of weight, culinary geniuses who are out to improve their unhappy lot are hard to take.

Making up the Calories

The diet used in conjunction with HCG must not exceed 500 calories per day, and the way these calories are made up is of utmost importance. For instance, if a patient drops the apple and eats an extra breadstick instead, he will not be getting more calories but he will not lose weight. There are a number of foods, particularly fruits and vegetables, which have the same or even lower caloric values than those listed as permissible, and yet we find that they interfere with the regular loss of weight under HCG, presumably owing to the nature of their composition. Pimiento peppers, okra, artichokes and pears are examples of this.

While this diet works satisfactorily in Italy, certain modifications have to be made in other countries. **For instance, American beef has almost double the caloric value of South Italian beef, which is not marbled with fat. This marbling is impossible to remove**. In America, therefore, low-grade veal should be used for one meal and fish (excluding all those species such as herring, mackerel, salmon, eel, etc., which have a high fat content, and all dried, smoked or pickled fish), chicken breast, lobster, crawfish, prawns or shrimp, crabmeat or kidneys for the other meal. Where the Italian breadsticks, the so-called grissini, are not available, one Melba toast may be used instead, though they are psychologically less satisfying. A Melba toast has about the same weight as the very porous grissini which is much more to look at and to chew.

When local conditions or the feeding habits of the population make changes necessary, it must be borne in mind that the total daily intake must not exceed 500 calories if the best possible results are to be obtained, and that the daily ration should contain 200 grams of fat-free protein and a very small amount of starch.

Just as the daily dose of HCG is the same in all cases, so the same diet proves to be satisfactory for a small elderly lady of leisure or a hard working muscular giant. "**Under the effect of HCG the obese body is always able to obtain all the calories it needs from the abnormal fat deposits, regardless of whether it uses up 1500 or 4000 calories per day. It must be made very clear to the patient that he is living to a far greater extent on the fat which he is losing than on what he eats.**"

Many patients ask why eggs are not allowed. The contents of two good sized eggs are roughly equivalent to 100 grams of meat, but unfortunately the yolk contains a large amount of fat, which is undesirable. Very occasionally we allow egg - boiled, poached or raw - to patients who develop an aversion to meat, but in this case they must add the white of three eggs to the one they eat whole. In countries where cottage cheese made from skimmed milk is available, 100 grams may occasionally be used instead of the meat, but no other cheeses are allowed.

Above Excerpt directly from Pounds and Inches: A New Approach to Obesity although a few mistakes have been corrected for ease of understanding.

Food Observations that may be of interest to new participants:

A few considerations on possible additional alternatives...

- Many participants have concluded that tuna was not allowed in the 1950s because all tuna was packed in oil at that time. Now that tuna is packed in water, participants have experimented and found that tuna appears to encourage rapid weight loss just like the other white fish that are allowed on the 500 calorie phase of the protocol.

- In the Midwest, many participants have experimented with venison (deer) for a couple of reasons: we doubt that Dr. Simeons tested venison since it is a wild meat, and venison is an extremely low fat meat. Accordingly, we can report that we have seen good, consistent weight loss with venison.

We do not suggest deviations from Dr. Simeons' list lightly. We have followed over a thousand participants from start to finish, as Dr. Simeons recommended, before noting any deviations such as the water-packed tuna and venison.

So, to be clear, we are quite confident that typical foods such as green beans, broccoli and turkey were all thoroughly tested by Dr. Simeons. Furthermore, since there has been no significant change in the handling of these common foods (like with the tuna being packed in water vs. oil), we surmise that these foods did not meet Dr. Simeons requirements for making the list and are, therefore, simply not acceptable. Of course, there are and will be participants who use these and other 'off-list' foods, but you should use great caution since these may SLOW your rate of loss or simply not fulfill the nutritional demands that Dr. Simeons required.

Summary of allowable 500 calorie diet foods (Phase 2)

With caloric values for those dieters who absolutely would not feel comfortable without more details:

Breakfast: Tea or coffee in any quantity – Only one tablespoonful of milk allowed per day
Saccharin, or stevia that does not have any invalid fillers

Lunch or Dinner:

(1) 100 grams of one lean meat or white fish (weighed raw); **Vary protein selection daily**

Grilled or baked (no oil or fat) allowed:

1).	Beef a) Steak	140 calories	
	b) Extra Lean Ground Beef	215 calories	
	c) Beef, Roast	150 calories	
2).	Buffalo	150 calories	
3).	Veal	110 calories	
4).	Chicken breast (skinless/boneless)	110 calories	
5).	Wild Chilean sea bass	120 calories	
6).	Wild flounder	110 calories	
7).	Wild sole	120 calories	
8).	Wild Halibut	110 calories	
9).	Lobster	95 calories	
10).	Crab	55 calories	
11).	Shrimp	90 calories	

(2) Vegetables: allowed **ONLY ONE** kind per meal **NO MIXING; Vary vegetable selection daily:**

1).	Lettuces of any kind	16 calories	2 cups
2).	Spinach	13 calories	2 cups
3).	Asparagus	62 calories	2 cups
4).	Cabbage	35 calories	2 cups
5).	Tomatoes	65 calories	1 cup
6).	Cucumbers	29 calories	2 cups
7).	Chard	14 calories	2 cups
8).	White, yellow or red onions	61 calories	1 cup
9).	Beet Greens	14 calories	2 cups
10).	Red radishes	46 calories	2 cups
11).	Celery	38 calories	2 cups
12).	Fennel	40 calories	1 1/2 cups
13).	Chicory greens	41 calories	1 cup

(3) Fruit: pick one per Lunch and Dinner

1).	Medium sized Apple	80 calories	
2).	Medium sized Orange	60 calories	
3).	1/2 medium sized Grapefruit	40 calories	
4).	Handful of organic Strawberries	35 calories	6-10 med 1-1/4in

(4) Breadstick grissini or Melba toast (one):

1.	Grissini Breadstick	20 calories
2.	Melba toast (round)	20 calories

Anything may be eliminated if desired per Dr. Simeons' manuscript as your body will be getting significant nutrients from the weight being released by the HCG. But remember to keep both body and mind healthy regarding food and eating. Prepare yourself physically and mentally for your future healthy lifestyle.

Seasonings Allowed: Salt, pepper, vinegar, mustard powder, garlic, sweet basil, parsley, thyme, marjoram, etc. The juice of one lemon daily is allowed for all purposes.

Drinks Allowed: Plain spring water, mineral water, tea, coffee, are the only drinks allowed, but they may be taken in any quantity and at all times. **You should drink about 2 liters of these fluids per day.**

HCG Protocol Friendly Products during the 500 Calorie Diet Phase

What hygiene / beauty care products can be used during the 500 calorie diet days of the HCG protocol?

Dr. Simeons wrote that "Most women find it hard to believe that fats, oils, creams, and ointments applied to the skin are absorbed and interfere with weight reduction by HCG just as if they had been eaten. This almost incredible sensitivity to even such very minor increases in nutritional intake is a peculiar feature of the HCG method."

Because of the system's 'incredible sensitivity' to sugars, starches, oils and fats, either put IN or ON the body, one should be vigilantly mindful of everything that goes into the mouth OR comes in contact with skin. If, for example, one must apply a healing ointment to a baby's diaper rash several times a day, gloves should be worn. If a person on HCG is cut and some type of antibiotic ointment is in order, apply a minimal amount and make note on your daily weight chart. Often times, the average person tends to apply far more product than necessary.

Dr. Simeons specified in the diet that "... no cosmetics other than lipstick, eyebrow pencil and powder may be used without special permission." However, in some cases, the modern day market is quite different than it was fifty years ago. At the time the good doctor composed his manuscript, mascara, for example, was made with petroleum jelly, which is most probably why it was not allowed, and almost all other cosmetic products had lanolin and oils as ingredients. Today there are many 'oil free' products available including foundation, sunscreen, and other makeup type products.

The following list contains some products used by some HCG participants without apparently slowing weight loss. If you have doubts about using a product, make note of what is used on your weight chart so that you can discern if certain products cause a stall or slow down in weight loss for you. For both healthy food and healthy products, retailers like Wild Oats and Whole Foods are great places to shop and ask questions.

The bottom line...Do you have to replace all your regular hygiene / makeup products with those listed in this book? NO! Analyze your personal hygiene habits and decide which product usage should be suspended during the low calorie phase of the diet – definitely all products with oils, for example.

So, on one hand, your toothpaste may list sorbitol as the first inactive ingredient. While sorbitol is a sugar alcohol used in sugar free foods, gums and mints, which are not allowed on the low calorie phase of the HCG protocol, the toothpaste is only in your mouth for a few minutes and isn't swallowed. Therefore, your continued use is probably fine, but you could try an alternative to remove any and all doubt about this daily activity. On the other hand, an oil-based foundation, or base that remains on your face all day long, should definitely be replaced.

To further complicate the issue, keep in mind that everyone is different, and that every product / brand is slightly different. So, even though a product may be oil-free, some other ingredient or chemical in that product may inhibit weight loss for some participants. Again, make notes on your daily weight log to assist you in determining if a particular product seems to stall or slow your weight loss.

Note: All '*' products are suspect. Some participants think these are acceptable; others disagree strongly – use sparingly and note on your chart to determine if these slow your weight loss. It is highly advisable to continue to note use of these products through your entire round because you may appear to be losing fine for the first 7–10 days and then stall out because of products. Good loss in the first 7–10 days is NOT an indicator that these products are not affecting your weight loss.

Product Category   Where to Find

Cosmetics
Powders HIGHLY recommended

Bare Escentuals	Mall boutiques, see website
Max Factor Pancake	Discount retail stores
Raw Minerals	Salons, spas, see website
Oil-free base/foundation*	Many brands now have oil-free lines

Deodorants

Baking Soda	Grocery stores
Crystalux Crystal Deodorant	Health food stores, some chains
Crystal Deodorant Stick	Health food stores, internet, some chains
Thai Deodorant Stick	Health food stores, internet

Face Soaps / Make-up Removers

Arbonne - All Botanical Based Skin Care* (some products; not all)	Independent beauty consultants
Neutrogena Oil Free Cream Cleanser*	Discount retail stores
Witch Hazel	Discount retail stores or drug stores

Hair Color
We haven't identified any treatments that are perfect. Regardless, many participants have used hair coloring treatments during the low calorie phase, and while they may have not lost weight that day, the treatment did not have an ongoing effect, and many didn't note any difference in weight loss.

Skin/Lip Moisturizers

Alba Oil Free Facial Moisturizer*	Discount retail stores
Aloe Vera 100% Gel	Discount retail stores or drug stores
Baby Oil (basically mineral oil)	Discount retail stores or drug stores
Coconut Oil* (Cold pressed, not expeller pressed)	Discount retail stores or drug stores
Corn Huskers Lotion*	Discount retail stores or drug stores
Curel Continuous Comfort, Fragrance Free*	Discount retail stores or drug stores
Fiji Organic Virgin Coconut Oil for Body, Massage & Hair*	Health food stores, internet
Kiss My Face Oil Free Moisturizer*	Specialty Store Chains, internet
Mineral Oil	Discount retail stores or drug stores
Neutrogena Oil Free Facial Lotion*	Discount retail stores or drug stores
St. Ives Vanilla Lotion*	Discount retail stores or drug stores
Zia Oil Free Body Lotion*	Health food stores, internet

Product Category	Where to Find

Shampoos/Conditioners

Aubrey Organics (some products; not all)	Health food stores, website
Fiji Organic Virgin Coconut Oil for Body, Massage & Hair	Health food stores, internet
Life Extension (some products; not all)	Health food stores, internet
Magik Botanicals Oil Free Shampoo & Conditioner	Internet
Mastey Products (some products; not all)	Beauty salons, internet
Natures Gate Alovera	Health food stores, internet

Soap

Baking Soda	Grocery stores
Dial	Discount retail stores or drug stores
Ivory	Discount retail stores or drug stores
Jason's	Health food stores, internet
Zest	Discount retail stores or drug stores

Sunscreen

Aveeno Oil Free Sunscreen*	Discount retail stores or drugstores
Clarins Oil Free Sun Care Spray SPF 15*	Department stores
Coppertone Oil Free Sun Block Lotion for Faces SPF 30*	Discount retail stores or drugstores
Coppertone Oil Free Sun Block Lotion*	Discount retail stores or drugstores
Ocean Potion Sport Extreme Sun Block Water & Sweat*	Discount retail stores or drugstores
Oil Free Sport Xtreme Sun Block*	Discount retail stores or drugstores
Peter Thomas Roth Ultra Lite Oil Free sun products*	Spas, department stores and internet
Zia Oil Free Sunscreen SPF 15*	Health food stores, internet

Toothpaste

Baking Soda	Grocery stores
Spry Toothpaste	Health food stores, internet
Tom's of Maine Toothpaste	Drug stores

Additional Hygiene & Beauty Care Products Information

Note: Pay the most attention to products that have oil and are rubbed into and quickly absorbed by the skin, such as lotion, liquid foundations, antibiotic creams (i.e. Neosporin, diaper rash ointments). And keep in mind that some of the products listed here are chosen more for better health benefits than for weight loss (i.e. Chrystal deodorant).

It is **not** necessary to buy most of these items to successfully lose weight. Most participants use their same deodorant, soap, shampoo, conditioner and toothpaste with great results. Most participants do use powder foundation OR avoid makeup for the low calorie diet days. Most participants avoid skin and lip moisturizers as much as possible. For extremely dry hands, participants report decent relief from applying baby oil and gloves before going to bed at night.

Sample Gorge Days
(Just ideas, don't make yourself sick.)

Breakfast: Cream cheese bagel with bacon and sausage, and a ham/cheese omelet.
Mid-morning snack: Donut with whipped cream and strawberries.
Lunch: Pork chop, potato with sour cream, a roll with butter and a buttered vegetable.
Mid-afternoon snack: ice cream (real) with Oreos and/or Twinkies.
Dinner: Fettuccini, cheese bread, and salad w/ regular dressing –don't forget cheesecake for dessert.
Late-night snack: Ice cream or frozen cappuccino.
Note: You can't go wrong by hitting your favorite fast food restaurant for an order of fries and a quarter pounder or donuts with a frozen coffee for those of us who don't like to make it ourselves.

Sample 500 Calorie Day Menu

Breakfast

Tea or coffee	5 calories
1 tablespoon 2% milk	8 calories

Lunch

1). Orange roughy (grilled), (100 grams weighed raw)	110 calories
2). Asparagus	30 calories 1 cup
3). Medium sized Apple	80 calories
4). Melba Toast	20 calories

Dinner

1). Steak (grilled), (100 grams weighed raw)	140 calories
2). Spinach	10 calories 1.5 cups
3). Strawberries	30 calories 7 med
4). Grissini Breadstick	20 calories
DAILY TOTAL CALORIES	453 CALORIES

Breakfast

Tea or coffee	5 calories

Lunch

1). Chicken breast (grilled), (100 grams weighed raw)	110 calories
2). Slaw (cabbage w/ vinegar, water, Stevia dressing)	40 calories
3). Medium sized Apple	80 calories
4). Grissini	20 calories

Dinner

1). Shrimp (grilled), (100 grams weighed raw)	110 calories
2). Lettuce w/apple cider vinegar, water, Stevia dressing	15 calories 1.5 cups
3). Orange	60 calories
4). Melba	20 calories
DAILY TOTAL CALORIES	460 CALORIES

Remember, you can eat up to 500 calories by making your choices, but you do not have to eat 500 calories, so do not 'back into' how much of anything you can eat. Make your selections and only look at calories to make sure you aren't exceeding the 500 for some reason.

Weekly Intake during 500 Calorie Phase Form

DAY 1 Weight ___

Breakfast
☐ Tea (any time
☐ Coffee (any time)

Miscellaneous
☐ 1 Tbsp Milk
☐ 1 Lemon

Lunch
Protein: ☐ Chicken ☐ Veal ☐ Lean Beef
☐ White fish/Seafood (what kind _____)
Fruit: ☐ Apple ☐ Grapefruit ☐ Strawberries
☐ Orange
Vegetable: _____
Breadstick: ☐ Grissino ☐ Melba Toast
Notes:_____

Dinner
Protein: ☐ Chicken ☐ Veal ☐ Lean Beef
☐ White fish/Seafood (what kind _____)
Fruit: ☐ Apple ☐ Grapefruit ☐ Strawberries
☐ Orange
Vegetable: _____
Breadstick: ☐ Grissino ☐ Melba Toast

DAY 2 Weight ___

Breakfast
☐ Tea (any time
☐ Coffee (any time)

Miscellaneous
☐ 1 Tbsp Milk
☐ 1 Lemon

Lunch
Protein: ☐ Chicken ☐ Veal ☐ Lean Beef
☐ White fish/Seafood (what kind _____)
Fruit: ☐ Apple ☐ Grapefruit ☐ Strawberries
☐ Orange
Vegetable: _____
Breadstick: ☐ Grissino ☐ Melba Toast
Notes:_____

Dinner
Protein: ☐ Chicken ☐ Veal ☐ Lean Beef
☐ White fish/Seafood (what kind _____)
Fruit: ☐ Apple ☐ Grapefruit ☐ Strawberries
☐ Orange
Vegetable: _____
Breadstick: ☐ Grissino ☐ Melba Toast

DAY 3 Weight ___

Breakfast
☐ Tea (any time
☐ Coffee (any time)

Miscellaneous
☐ 1 Tbsp Milk
☐ 1 Lemon

Lunch
Protein: ☐ Chicken ☐ Veal ☐ Lean Beef
☐ White fish/Seafood (what kind _____)
Fruit: ☐ Apple ☐ Grapefruit ☐ Strawberries
☐ Orange
Vegetable: _____
Breadstick: ☐ Grissino ☐ Melba Toast
Notes:_____

Dinner
Protein: ☐ Chicken ☐ Veal ☐ Lean Beef
☐ White fish/Seafood (what kind _____)
Fruit: ☐ Apple ☐ Grapefruit ☐ Strawberries
☐ Orange
Vegetable: _____
Breadstick: ☐ Grissino ☐ Melba Toast

DAY 4 Weight ___

Breakfast
☐ Tea (any time
☐ Coffee (any time)

Miscellaneous
☐ 1 Tbsp Milk
☐ 1 Lemon

Lunch
Protein: ☐ Chicken ☐ Veal ☐ Lean Beef
☐ White fish/Seafood (what kind _____)
Fruit: ☐ Apple ☐ Grapefruit ☐ Strawberries
☐ Orange
Vegetable: _____
Breadstick: ☐ Grissino ☐ Melba Toast
Notes:_____

Dinner
Protein: ☐ Chicken ☐ Veal ☐ Lean Beef
☐ White fish/Seafood (what kind _____)
Fruit: ☐ Apple ☐ Grapefruit ☐ Strawberries
☐ Orange
Vegetable: _____
Breadstick: ☐ Grissino ☐ Melba Toast

DAY 5 Weight ___

Breakfast
☐ Tea (any time
☐ Coffee (any time)

Miscellaneous
☐ 1 Tbsp Milk
☐ 1 Lemon

Lunch
Protein: ☐ Chicken ☐ Veal ☐ Lean Beef
☐ White fish/Seafood (what kind _____)
Fruit: ☐ Apple ☐ Grapefruit ☐ Strawberries
☐ Orange
Vegetable: _____
Breadstick: ☐ Grissino ☐ Melba Toast
Notes:_____

Dinner
Protein: ☐ Chicken ☐ Veal ☐ Lean Beef
☐ White fish/Seafood (what kind _____)
Fruit: ☐ Apple ☐ Grapefruit ☐ Strawberries
☐ Orange
Vegetable: _____
Breadstick: ☐ Grissino ☐ Melba Toast

DAY 6 Weight ___

Breakfast
☐ Tea (any time
☐ Coffee (any time)

Miscellaneous
☐ 1 Tbsp Milk
☐ 1 Lemon

Lunch
Protein: ☐ Chicken ☐ Veal ☐ Lean Beef
☐ White fish/Seafood (what kind _____)
Fruit: ☐ Apple ☐ Grapefruit ☐ Strawberries
☐ Orange
Vegetable: _____
Breadstick: ☐ Grissino ☐ Melba Toast
Notes:_____

Dinner
Protein: ☐ Chicken ☐ Veal ☐ Lean Beef
☐ White fish/Seafood (what kind _____)
Fruit: ☐ Apple ☐ Grapefruit ☐ Strawberries
☐ Orange
Vegetable: _____
Breadstick: ☐ Grissino ☐ Melba Toast

DAY 7 Weight ___

Breakfast
☐ Tea (any time
☐ Coffee (any time)

Miscellaneous
☐ 1 Tbsp Milk
☐ 1 Lemon

Lunch
Protein: ☐ Chicken ☐ Veal ☐ Lean Beef
☐ White fish/Seafood (what kind _____)
Fruit: ☐ Apple ☐ Grapefruit ☐ Strawberries
☐ Orange
Vegetable: _____
Breadstick: ☐ Grissino ☐ Melba Toast
Notes:_____

Dinner
Protein: ☐ Chicken ☐ Veal ☐ Lean Beef
☐ White fish/Seafood (what kind _____)
Fruit: ☐ Apple ☐ Grapefruit ☐ Strawberries
☐ Orange
Vegetable: _____
Breadstick: ☐ Grissino ☐ Melba Toast

Most Common Errors during 500 Calorie Diet Phase

1. **Using the wrong spices**. Spices must be used with extreme caution. Check all ingredients for any unallowable foods (shredded orange peel), any form of sugar (brown, white, maltose, dextrose, etc,), starch (modified corn starch), and/or any kind of oil i.e. 'Garlic Salt' can have sugar and modified cornstarch—not acceptable!

2. **Not loading enough fat** during load (gorge) days (first two days of HCG). This might explain hunger and associated crankiness during the first week of HCG low calorie phase.

3. **Mixing vegetables at a meal**. Dr. Simeons clearly states one vegetable. While many people lose quite satisfactorily when mixing vegetables, it is a place to review if losing slows.

4. **Chewing gum, mints, etc**. These items are not allowed during the VLCD (very low calorie diet phase). Again, some lose quite satisfactorily when violating this directive, but it is a place to review if losing slows.

5. **Drinking unallowed diet drinks** including Crystal Light, diet soda or other diet drinks – only water, teas, coffees, and mineral water should be used. Use allowable, flavored stevia in your water, coffee and tea for extra flavor and variety. Note: Carbonated water is not recommended.

6. **Eating too much American, ground beef**, which is noted as significantly more fatty than the beef Dr. Simeons refers to. Veal is a possible suggested replacement. Buffalo can be less fatty than American beef and is available at Trader Joe's at this time. Many participants can quicken weight loss by eating less beef and more chicken or allowable fish/seafood, in particular.

7. **Weighing 100 grams of protein *after* cooking**. Weight of protein is to be based on PRECOOKED weight– this can make quite a difference in the prescribed serving.

8. **Eating the same protein for both lunch and dinner**. Food selections are to be varied.

9. **Not drinking enough water.** You should be drinking at least 2 quarts of water and other allowable liquids per day.

10. **Weighing in significantly different clothes** or at different times each morning (before eating or drinking) causes undue concern and confusion or false appearance of weight gain/loss.

11. **Eating at restaurants**. To a large degree the meats have been 'juiced' or manipulated to be more flavorful, tender or juicy, with a multitude of processes that could easily slow your weight loss, particularly chicken.

12. **Using moisturizers, eye creams,** night creams, makeup removers and other products on the skin. Dr. Simeons warned of the extreme sensitivity experienced while HCG is in the body.

Most Common Concerns during the 500 Calorie Phase (P2)

1. **Constipation** can be a concern. Many people find relief with Green tea or Smooth Move Tea. Some participants report that adding Apricot Nectar stevia to water is quite effective for staying regular also.

2. **Hair loss** is a scary concern. Two very important points follow:
    a. **To date, no one has reported losing all of their hair.**
    b. **Everyone has reported that their hair grows back.**

   Obviously, these points are important because hair loss is very concerning, and these points may make the difference between continuing the protocol and stopping. For example, losing hair may be terrifying, but if you are quite sure that it will grow back, you are much more likely to continue the HCG protocol.

   Many sources would have you believe that hair loss either during or after the HCG cycle means that the HCG protocol is completely unhealthy and directly causing hair loss. You should be aware that many woman experience significant hair loss after having a baby, after losing significant weight with any diet method, or after stopping hormones or other medications.

   Hair loss typically tapers off and then grows back without any intervention, but burdock root tea can be used to help the process along. (Pour hot water over a couple of tea bags of burdock root tea bags, allow it to sit overnight, warm up one time in the morning, then pour it on your scalp or spray it in your hair like leave-in conditioner and comb through after you shower in the morning. Make a new batch every 4-5 days). Thymuskin shampoo and treatment has also been mentioned as a successful solution. The forums listed in this book and other HCG forums offer many suggestions for hair loss. Note: We have seen less reports of hair loss with the Homeopathic HCG.

3. **Leg cramps** during sleep are not common. However, for the participants who experience leg cramps, the occurrence can be quite frequent and quite painful. Some tricks to avoid leg cramps are to avoid asparagus (a natural diuretic that may contribute to low potassium) and to increase your intake of spinach/chard as these vegetables are high in potassium. Another deficiency that can cause leg cramps is iron. While both iron and potassium are available in supplemental form, you should use caution and consider consulting with your physician, because too much iron or potassium can cause other serious issues. One other note, when you take iron, you may want to take vitamin C at the same time to assist in absorbency per some physicians' advice.

   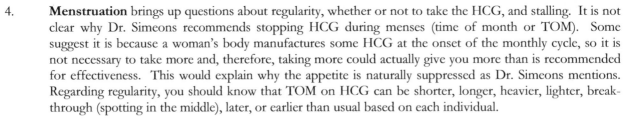

   Note: We have seen significantly less leg cramps when Homeopathic Cell Salts (see photo to the right) are taken during the VLCD. If the cell salts are homeopathic, they have no nutritional value. Some brands of Homeopathic HCG have cell salts in the HCG, such as Pounds and Inches Away Advanced HCG Formula and DIY HCG brand.

4. **Menstruation** brings up questions about regularity, whether or not to take the HCG, and stalling. It is not clear why Dr. Simeons recommends stopping HCG during menses (time of month or TOM). Some suggest it is because a woman's body manufactures some HCG at the onset of the monthly cycle, so it is not necessary to take more and, therefore, taking more could actually give you more than is recommended for effectiveness. This would explain why the appetite is naturally suppressed as Dr. Simeons mentions. Regarding regularity, you should know that TOM on HCG can be shorter, longer, heavier, lighter, break-through (spotting in the middle), later, or earlier than usual based on each individual.

   Regarding whether or not to take the HCG during menses, since Dr. Simeons takes the time to mention this subject several times, why not try following his advice of stopping the HCG during menses. **If you run into trouble with hunger, you can always decide to restart the HCG at any time**. There are plenty of participants who stop HCG the whole time, some who stop on heavy days, some who stop the first two days, and some who don't stop at all, but take the HCG straight through. Finally, if you stall or even have slight gains during this time, it is probably due to water retention assuming you are strictly following the protocol. Simply keep going – do not give up for a couple of days or cheat, which could actually cause a 'real' gain in weight. The water weight will fall off and you will continue on your way.

Tips and Hints for Success during the 500 Calorie Phase (P2)

Time Saving Tips

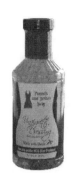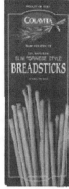

➢ Check out HCG protocol-friendly websites for great ideas and recipes. Additionally, more and more HCG protocol approved products are becoming available for your convenience on websites like: www.HCGPerfectPortions.com. Grocery items that are designed for the HCG Protocol can save quite a bit of time, i.e. the Vinaigrette Dressing (see photo to the right) is great on salads, vegetables, and as a marinade for meats; which are also available in pre-portioned 3.5 oz. steak, veal, and ground beef selections. Stevia, both plain and flavored, and grissini breadsticks are offered as well.

➢ Purchase thawed protein servings (shrimp, chicken breast, crab, and fish) and, instead of putting it in the freezer in big quantities, divides the portions into the prescribed 100 gram servings, then freeze in individual size servings. Note: Some participants take this one step further and actually cook the protein before freezing so that it can just be reheated or put on a salad before eating.

➢ Each morning (or the night before) pick two different proteins for the upcoming day and move them to the refrigerator to thaw. Thawing won't take long and cooking only takes a couple of minutes on the George Foreman grill. This saves quite a bit of time compared to freezing large packages of frozen chicken breasts, etc. and trying to work with these packages when you want your 100 grams for a meal.

➢ Fill 7-14 syringes at a time instead of one every morning if using the HCG Injections.

➢ Use a George Foreman grill for meat – almost everything is done in about 3 minutes.

➢ Make some chicken broth using the recipe in the 101 Worry – Free HCG Recipe Book or a similar recipe as soon as you start the protocol. This broth can then be used for a soup base and to cook your vegetables.

Tasty Tips

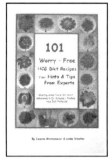

➢ Pickup the "101 Worry-Free HCG Diet Recipes" book (see photo to the right), this book has enough variety to get you through a HCG cycle without getting bored with the food.

➢ Dressing for lettuce, cucumbers, tomatoes, onions, cabbage/slaw: 1/3 c apple cider vinegar, 2/3 - 1 c water (to your taste preference), sweeten with stevia (takes pretty much to taste like dressing), salt and pepper to taste. Prepackaged dressing is available at www.HCGPerfectPortions.com.

➢ If your meat cooked on the George Foreman gets too dried out, use sweet, small Vidalia onions for your vegetable and throw them on the top and bottom of the meat on the grill. Both the meat and the onions are great!

➢ Add more teas to your diet. Some teas cleanse the body, some increase your metabolism and some just taste like a treat, but watch all ingredients carefully. If the ingredients list any fruit, oil, vegetable, etc., do not use the tea during the low-calorie phase.

➢ Condiments such as plain yellow mustard and some brands of hot sauce can be utilized to add flavor and spice to your meals. Make sure there isn't any sugar in the ingredients. Use with caution, because these can stall or slow loss for some participants.

➢ Some people have found success substituting a dill pickle for the cucumber serving. Don't choose any pickles that have oils, starches, or sugars i.e. fructose corn syrup listed in the ingredients and monitor weight closely.

➢ MMM…MMM…fresh squeezed lemonade -- I have personally made 3 large glasses of lemonade with one juicy lemon and plenty of stevia packets, which took me through an entire night at the stadium.

➢ Cut an apple in half, sprinkle with stevia and cinnamon and microwave for approximately 2 minutes.

➢ Coffee with allowed milk plus stevia, cinnamon and a couple drops of pure vanilla extract is very close to a real flavored coffee

➢ Stevia comes in many flavors: Grape, Cinnamon, Vanilla Creme, English Toffee, Berry, Valencia Orange, Lemon Drop, Chocolate Raspberry, Root Beer, Hazelnut and more.

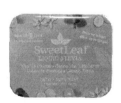
Stevia Travel Tin – 4 Flavors

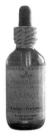
Clear Liquid Stevia

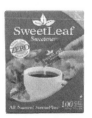
Stevia Packets

Plateau Breakers and Daily Loss Rate Maximizers (P2)

If your weight loss slows or stalls, don't panic. Do review the 'plateau' section of Dr. Simeons' manuscript in the Appendix of this guide. If you are cheating, your fix is easy – stop cheating. If you don't think you are doing anything wrong, review the most common errors list and consider some of the following ideas. Keep in mind that plateaus are not uncommon, and if you stick to the protocol they WILL pass. Some stalls can be explained (i.e. old weight set points, time of month, ovulation, steroids, sunburn), other plateaus cannot be explained, but all will pass if you stick to the protocol. The following ideas can help you both psychologically and physically make it through the slow times.

➢ Increase water intake to 2 - 3 quarts per day.

➢ Try adding a glass or two of green tea to your day.

➢ Don't eat 2 apples for the two fruits or cut down on the size of the apples.

➢ Cut American, ground, beef and/or buffalo down or out.

➢ Consider that oranges, tomatoes and shrimp stall **some** people. Therefore, if you eat either oranges, tomatoes, and/or shrimp quite a bit and your weight loss is slow, you may want to try cutting these foods down or out to see if your rate of loss increases. You may not be affected by some or all of these, so you should check one food at a time. To test yourself for sensitivity (slowed weight loss), have only one of the foods three days in a row, then repeat those three days' menus changing only the one food being tested. Compare the average weight loss from the first three days to the second three days. If there is no difference, consider the food safe. If there is a significant difference, drop the food that caused the sensitivity.

➢ Check all condiments for any form of sugar. 'Garlic Salt' may list sugar as an ingredient. Any seasoning salt or seasoning product must be carefully checked.

➢ If mixing vegetables, stop.

➢ If having trouble with constipation, try Green tea or Smooth Move tea.

➢ Try leaving out one or both breadsticks.

➢ Make sure there are no additives in chicken or other protein sources – many times these are injected with some form of sugar even in the grocery store.

➢ Consider the potency of your HCG – you may need new HCG. With Injection HCG and Mixed Sublingual HCG, potency can be checked by drawing up a bit of your mixed HCG and putting it on a pregnancy test kit that you would put urine on. This is not an accurate check for Homeopathic HCG – see FAQ for a full explanation. Potency of any HCG type can be affected by extreme temperatures, and other conditions.

➢ If using injections, consider if immunity could be setting in based on how long you have been taking shots (longer than 30 days), consider dosage (between 125 and 200), and whether a day per week has been skipped. Immunity is not as much an issue with Homeopathic HCG.

➢ Consider if you are potentially at your ideal weight. Are you in the suggested weight range for your height and build? Are you also hungry and not feeling as good, etc? It may be time to stop losing. See the manuscript for details on reaching your goal during a cycle of shots. Basically, you increase food intake to level off losing until the minimum number of shots is reached, then follow the protocol through the 6 week stabilizing/maintenance phase.

➢ For women, your cycle may be coming into play -- review Dr. Simeons' manuscript.

➤ Have you changed or started one or more medications? The change may just cause a few days delay as your body adjusts, but you may want to consult with your physician to possibly change again or go back to the previous medication if the plateau continues and all plateau breaking methods fail.

➤ Review the manuscript for serious plateaus (5 days or longer). While the manuscript reports 'apple days' as purely psychological, many participants report a loss of 2 pounds the day after an apple day.

➤ Since the protocol says you are not required to eat all the food each day, you may consider dropping one or both of the 'breads' and/or one of your fruits, etc.

➤ One client is not very hungry and likes to do a 'mini steak day' ever so often. If you are familiar with the manuscript, a 'steak day' refers to a routine you follow after you have completed the HCG phase and are weighing daily. During this time, if your morning weight is 2 pounds over your last HCG weight, you have a 'steak day'. A 'steak day' means you drink water, tea, and coffee when you want and in whatever quantity you want, but you do not eat anything until dinner. For dinner you have a large steak and either a raw tomato or an apple. So for a 'mini steak day', the client drinks allowable drinks, but basically has a 100 gram steak serving with an apple for dinner. That's it until the next day when she returns to the normal 500 diet. Again, the client does this when weight loss is stalled and she simply doesn't feel hungry anyway (obviously because the HCG is working so well).

➤ Consider adding a brisk walk, some yoga, or any type of 15 minute activities to your day a few times a week--anything that raises the heart rate throughout the day, but not muscle-building exercise if you are not use to it. The activity increases your metabolism and may increase your rate of loss. Exercise is barely mentioned in the protocol. Our interpretation is that exercise is good for everyone; however, it is simply not required to successfully lose weight on this protocol. That being said, we have observed participants who have a physically active job, such as a waitress, where the participant seemed to maintain a slightly higher daily average weight loss than those who did absolutely no physical activity.

➤ Make sure you are getting enough sleep. More than a few participants have reported being up late and getting up early and the scale reflecting little to no weight loss. However, simply weighing again an hour or so later (without eating or drinking anything) reveals a drop on the scale of up to 2 pounds. This suggests that routine and adequate sleep can effect what the scale registers.

➤ Try including 2 Tbsp of apple cider vinegar (ACV) to your daily regimen. Some resources recommend that you take the ACV diluted with water or juice, but not to spread out throughout the entire day as this has been shown to have negative effects on teeth enamel. Many resources claim extensive benefits due to (ACV) intake, particularly increased weight loss; however ACV may cause you discomfort if you digest the vinegar using undiluted spoonfuls only.

➤ If you are using tanning beds, consider stopping to see if it makes a difference.

Maintenance (P3 or Phase 3 as referenced in Trudeau's book)
The Philosophy

If you reach the maintenance phase, congratulations are in order. Successfully completing the HCG protocol is a feat to be proud of. The maintenance phase should be a well-deserved break during which your body and mind catch up with each other. Most participants have a strong feeling of accomplishment and overall well-being at this point. If you are tempted to not go to maintenance after 40 days of HCG because you have lost so well, do **NOT** give in to the temptation. Your body and mind need the break for many reasons including the avoidance of sagging skin and rebuilding your nutritional stockpiles. Dr. Simeons worked with the protocol for decades for best overall results – don't underestimate the purpose behind each step.

On one hand, maintenance should build on the success of the 500 calorie diet phase and give you additional confidence as you go on to a future HCG cycle or go on with life. On the other hand, the switch to the maintenance phase can be the biggest challenge of the entire HCG protocol. The maintenance phase is also known as Phase 3 or P3 from Kevin Trudeau's *The Weight Loss Cure "They" Don't Want You to Know About*.

Keep in mind, your goal during this phase is to maintain your new weight loss, not to lose more weight. If you have more weight to lose, you can do another round in 6 weeks (or more if this is not your first round; refer to Dr. Simeons Manuscript).

- o **YOUR GOAL:** To create a new weight set point, a weight that your body automatically maintains, close to your last HCG date weight.
- o **YOUR BODY'S GOAL:** To 'recover' the weight you lost. (This is what most people are unaware of when they 'finish' a diet.) Without a method to create a new weight set point, most bodies successfully 'recover' the lost weight – sound familiar?
- o To ensure that **YOUR GOAL** wins over **YOUR BODY'S GOAL**, you must perform the maintenance phase diligently.

Following is a Summary of Dr. Simeons' maintenance phase:

Eat what you want, when you want (preferably when you are hungry, and listen to your **body for** when you have had enough) except no sugars and no starches, and weigh EVERYDAY. If you are 2.1 pounds over your last injection (HCG) weight, perform a Steak Day*.

*Steak Day: "Skip breakfast and lunch but take plenty to drink. In the evening, eat a huge steak with only an apple or a raw tomato." Dr. Simeons

Be aware that the longer time you spend in a very small weight range, the better and quicker your body will settle in on your new weight set point. There are two main ideas that you should understand to be successful in locking in your new weight.

If you are 'bad' on the weekends and gain 3 - 5 pounds, and then you are 'good' during the weeks and lose the 3 – 5 pounds with strict dieting or steak days, you will **not** set your new weight. Then, when you stop manually controlling your weight with strict dieting or steak days, your body will automatically take you back to your last set point, which could be the point where you started the protocol. Understanding this is critical. On the other hand, as long as you are following the maintenance directives (No Sugar/No Starch), the small variances in weight, due to water retention or eating at a restaurant, should not hinder you from settling on your new weight set point.

For the calorie conscience participants, Dr. Simeons' rule may be too vague. Please note that most participants are successful going immediately to a daily intake of 1500 calories with the correct foods (no bad-for-you sugars or starches) because of the following calculation:

- HCG releases about 1500 - 4000 calories per day into your system (per Dr. Simeons' manuscript) + 500 calories you are eating on VLCD = 2000 - 4500 calories per day.
- So, to come off the VLCD (very low calorie diet) and enter maintenance (P3) with less than 1500 calories may be seriously cutting the number of calories your body has been using every day with the HCG. Therefore, your body may kick in to starvation mode.
- For example, if you go from 2000 calories (on HCG) to even 1200 calories, you have not increased by 700 calories (1200 calories on maintenance – 500 calories on HCG); instead you have decreased by 800 (2000 calories on HCG – 1200 calories on maintenance), sending your body back into the starvation metabolism that got you here in the first place. This is very difficult mentally for many life time dieters, so understanding is critical.

After being on the very low calorie phase of the HCG protocol, the maintenance phase should feel like the sky is the limit. Try not to get hung up on what you can't have (sugars and starches), but instead focus on what you can eat (pork chops, broccoli, turkey, almonds, etc.). The best plan of action is to 'protein up', enjoy some 'good-for-you' fats, eat lots of fresh fruits and a variety of vegetables. You should have caution with dairy, nuts and starchy vegetables, and simply enjoy P3 (maintenance). It is good to know that many people never 'need' a steak day, but you can have steak when you like. Keep in mind that the participants who had the most trouble were not eating enough, in general, and not enough protein especially. Protein seems to be a key in locking in and maintaining your new weight. Refer to **General Outline of Beverage/Food Items** in this guide to help with the food choices on the Maintenance (P3) and all phases of the HCG diet protocol.

Also, remember that **many** participants need to eat a MINIMUM of 1500 calories--by all means not the maximum to maintain their new weight. You are setting up your system for the future (while staying within 2 pounds of your LIW (last injection weight)) or last HCG weight. For example, most people do NOT want to be able to eat ONLY 1500 calories a day in the future. Eating less calories than your system is willing to handle may encourage your system to require less, which in turn would support less calories as you move into the future.

It can be scary entering the maintenance phase because you go from knowing exactly what to do and when to do it, to **Dr. Simeons' one rule: "eat what you want when you are hungry except NO sugars and NO starches**, but weigh every morning to make sure you stay within 2 pounds of weight as of last injection. If you do go over the 2 pound limit, perform a Steak Day."

NOTE: You should review advice from Dr. Simeons' manuscript as you near the end of the 500 calorie phase, particularly the following paragraphs: Concluding a Course, Skipping a Meal, Trouble after Treatment, Beware of Over-Enthusiasm, and Protein Deficiency.

Sample Maintenance Menus (Phase 3)

1st 3 weeks of Maintenance (P3) Sample Menu

In case you are not comfortable just going 'freestyle' into the maintenance phase, following the 'eat what you want except No sugar and No starch' rule, we have listed a sample base menu to get you started. This allows you to build confidence and not waste a lot of time worrying about every ounce of variance on the scale. The following sample menu works well with most participants. If you don't like something, any entry could be changed to foods you do like as long as you don't add sugars or starches when they are not allowed (during the first three weeks of maintenance).

Remember: NO Sugars and NO Starches for the 1st 3 Weeks of Maintenance

	Sample Day 1	Sample Day 2	Sample Day 3	Sample Day 4
Breakfast:	• 2 Eggs • Vidalia Onion cooked in Olive Oil • Cantaloupe	• 2 Eggs w/ Turkey Sausage & onions • Coffee w/ Creamer & Stevia	• Cottage Cheese w/ Fruit or Cinnamon, Sweetened w/ Stevia	• 2 Eggs w/ Green Peppers, Onions & Ham • Plum
Mid-morning snack:	• Apple w/ Peanut Butter	• Organic Fruit & Nut Trail Mix	• Serving of Pecans	• Organic Trail Mix
Lunch:	• Chicken Breast w/ Grilled Onions • Small Salad w/ REGULAR Dressing	• Hamburger Patty & Pickles w/ Ketchup • Small Salad w/ REGULAR Dressing	• Tuna Salad w/ Tomatoes on Lettuce • REGULAR Dressing	• Ham w/ Green Beans • Small Salad w/ REGULAR Dressing
Mid-afternoon snack:	• Organic Fruit & Nut Trail Mix	• Serving of Almonds	• Organic Trail Mix	• Apple w/ Peanut Butter
Dinner:	• Scallops • Cauliflower • Salad w/ REGULAR Dressing	• Turkey • Broccoli w/ a little melted Cheese • Salad w/REGULAR Dressing	• Grilled or Fried Pork Chops • Green Beans • Salad w/ REGULAR Dressing	• Steak • Broccoli • Salad w/ REGULAR Dressing
Late-night snack:	• Nectarine w/ Sugar Free Yogurt	• Apple w/ Peanut Butter	• Peach w/ Brie or Cream Cheese	• Almonds • Strawberries • Brie Cheese

2nd 3 weeks of Maintenance (P3) Sample Menu

"Slowly" is the key word to moving in to the later phases with success. It is absolutely imperative that you weigh daily and perform a "steak day" on the very day you weigh more than 2 pounds over your last HCG day or last injections day

Remember: Slowly Add Sugars and Starches for the 2nd 3 weeks of Maintenance

	Sample Day 1	Sample Day 2	Sample Day 3	Sample Day 4
Breakfast:	• 2 Eggs • Vidalia Onion cooked in Olive Oil • Cantaloupe	• Kashi Cereal • ½ Cup Milk • Grapes	• 2 Eggs w/ Onion, Green Peppers, & Mushrooms • Canadian Bacon	• Shredded Wheat Cereal • ½ Cup milk • Strawberries
Mid-morning snack:	• Apple w/ Peanut Butter	• Almonds	• Cheese Cubes or Sticks	• Sugar-Free/Fat-Free Pudding
Lunch:	• Hamburger w/ Cheese, Mayo, Ketchup & Pickle • Grilled Onions • Small Salad w/ REGULAR Dressing	• Chicken Breast w/ Grilled Onions • Small Salad w/ REGULAR Dressing	• Chef Salad w/ REGULAR Dressing	• Hot Wings • Small Salad w/ REGULAR Dressing
Mid-afternoon snack:	• Organic Trail Mix	• Apple w/ Peanut Butter	• Pork Rinds	• Peanuts
Dinner:	• Steak • ½ Potato w/ Sour Cream • Green Beans • Small Salad w/ REGULAR Dressing	• Scallops • Cauliflower • Salad w/ REGULAR Dressing • Slice of Garlic Bread	• Polish Sausage • Saur Kraut • Small Serving of Mashed Potatoes	• Chicken Fajita w/ Grilled Peppers & Onions • Shredded Cheese • Refried Beans • Low-Carb Tortilla
Late-night snack:	• Almonds • Strawberries • Brie Cheese	• Tuna Salad scooped w/ Celery Sticks	• Apple w/ Peanut Butter	• Cottage Cheese w/ Real Fruit

Healthy, Safe Maintenance Snacks (P3)

Fruits

Vegetables

Edamame (young soybeans)

Celery with cheese* or peanut butter*

Apple with peanut butter*

Cottage cheese with real fruit

Beef Jerky (most flavors, but watch the sugars)

Turkey Jerky

Pork Rinds

Venison/Deer Jerky

Almonds*

Peanuts*

Cheese cubes/sticks*

Celery filled with tuna or chicken salad

Dessert-like Snacks

Sugar-free Fat-free Jell-o

Sugar-free Fat-free Pudding

Berries with Fat-free milk or Cream

Strawberries with Brie Cheese*

Skinny Cow Skinny Dippers*

*These items are caution items for the 1st 3 weeks of maintenance. Eat these in moderation and watch your morning weight closely.

Combination Food Snacks i.e. Snack Bars, Trail Mixes/Granola, Yogurt (P3)

Combination foods that make good, healthy snacks generally should be:

Carbohydrates 20 or less   **Fiber** 2 or more   **Sugar** 10 or less   **Protein** 4 or more

Some of the higher sugar examples below made the list because some of the 'sugar' is from the real fruit in the snack, so it is different than regular sugar.

Note: The *less* carbs/sugar grams, the better. The *more* fiber/protein grams, the better.

Snack Bars:

Pure Protein-High Protein Bars Chocolate Deluxe (Carb 17, Fiber 2, Sugar 2, Protein 20)*

South Beach Diet – High Protein Cereal Bars (Average: Carb 15, Fiber 3, Sugar 7, Protein 10)*

True North Pecan Almond Peanut Clusters (Carb 9, Fiber 2, Sugar 5, Protein, 5)*

Trio bars (Carb 14, Fiber 2, Sugar 6, Protein 5)*

Trail Mixes/Granola:

Planters Trail Mix Energy Mix (Carb 14, Fiber 3, Sugar 6, Protein 6)*

Slim Fast High Protein – Peanut Granola (Carb 20, Fiber 2, Sugar 10*, Protein 15) – Caution *

Ksar Pistachios – Sahale Snacks Nut Blend (Carb 11, Fiber 3, Sugar 3, Protein 5)*

Deerfield Farms – Snackin' Flax Granola Bites w/Cranberries, Blueberries & Raisins (Carb 20, Fiber 3, Sugar 8, Protein 4)*

Trader Joe's Organic Almonds, Cashews, and Cranberries Mix (Carb 15, Fiber 5, Sugar 8, Protein 9)*

Trader Joe's – San Wasabi Peas (Carb 19, Fiber 1, Sugar 2, Protein 4)*

Yogurt:

Dannon Light & Fit Carb & Sugar Control (Carb 3, Fiber 0, Sugar 2, Protein 5)*

Fiber One Creamy Non-Fat Yogurt (Carb 19, Fiber 5, Sugar 11, Protein 4)*

*These items are caution items for the 1st 3 weeks of maintenance. Eat these in moderation and watch your morning weight closely.

Weekly Intake During Maintenance Form

This is a (check one):   ☐ NO Sugars and NO Starch week (weeks 1 - 3 after end of HCG)

                         ☐ SLOWLY add Sugars/Starches week (weeks 4 - 6 after end of HCG)

DAY 1 Weight _____   **Lunch**   **Dinner**
Breakfast   _____   _____
_____   _____   _____
_____   _____   _____

Drinks and Snacks throughout the day: _____
_____

DAY 2 Weight _____   **Lunch**   **Dinner**
Breakfast   _____   _____
_____   _____   _____
_____   _____   _____

Drinks and Snacks throughout the day: _____
_____

DAY 3 Weight _____   **Lunch**   **Dinner**
Breakfast   _____   _____
_____   _____   _____
_____   _____   _____

Drinks and Snacks throughout the day: _____
_____

DAY 4 Weight _____   **Lunch**   **Dinner**
Breakfast   _____   _____
_____   _____   _____
_____   _____   _____

Drinks and Snacks throughout the day: _____
_____

DAY 5 Weight _____   **Lunch**   **Dinner**
Breakfast   _____   _____
_____   _____   _____
_____   _____   _____

Drinks and Snacks throughout the day: _____
_____

DAY 6 Weight _____   **Lunch**   **Dinner**
Breakfast   _____   _____
_____   _____   _____
_____   _____   _____

Drinks and Snacks throughout the day: _____
_____

DAY 7 Weight _____   **Lunch**   **Dinner**
Breakfast   _____   _____
_____   _____   _____
_____   _____   _____

Drinks and Snacks throughout the day: _____
_____

Weekly Notes: _____

If you have trouble locking-in your weight on maintenance, this form should be meticulously completed every day. Memory is simply not accurate enough to problem solve and this would provide your intake as weekly snapshots to analyze what is working for you and what isn't.

Tips and Hints for Success during the Maintenance Phase (P3)

➢ The maintenance phase of the HCG protocol is NOT the Atkins diet. The major differences are that you can eat most fruits and vegetables whenever you like AND you are not encouraged to consistently eat foods with high fat content. Remember, you are training your new body to maintain your new weight – eat healthier to feel better, look better, and successfully lock-in your new weight.

➢ Try to include protein throughout your day including meals and snacks. Good snack examples are listed on the next page.

➢ When picking snacks, you should pay more attention to sugar (other than natural sugar in fruit), than fat.

➢ Eat REAL food: real fruits, real fats (olive oil, almonds, regular salad dressing, and real cream), and real meat (seafood, pork, chicken, hot wings, fish).

➢ Avoid restaurants, but don't overreact if you are up a pound or two after eating at a restaurant since it is probably water retention if you followed the no sugar, no starch rule.

➢ Avoid processed lunch meat, canned fruits and canned vegetables; go for raw, minimally cooked, and frozen as much as possible.

➢ Avoid food and drinks that have many ingredients that you can't even pronounce.

➢ Continue to drink plenty of water – it is good for you and helps your body function efficiently.

➢ When buying packages of organic fruit and nut trail mix, almonds and other snack type food, divide into single serving sizes immediately upon arriving home from the store. These are conveniently stored in small zipper sandwich bags. This step helps you monitor how much you are eating in case you need to adjust due to weight gain/loss.

➢ If you struggle to maintain your loss, keep a food journal while you try to help your body and metabolism lock-in to this new weight for the next 6 or so weeks (in case you are doing another cycle) or forever because you reached your goal weight (Congratulations!). This will help identify your personal trouble foods. A sample journal is included for your convenience.

➢ For most participants, protein need not be watched carefully, while dairy and higher carbohydrate fruits and vegetables should be watched very carefully. Dr. Simeons warns about the very sweet fruits (may include melons, grapes, pineapple, bananas). Vegetables to avoid are potatoes, corn, peas, etc., but you should also be careful with most beans (other than string beans) like pinto, black, lima, etc. as these are starchier than most vegetables.

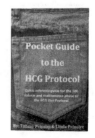

➢ Utilize the quick reference for the maintenance phase of the HCG diet protocol in the *Pocket Guide to the HCG Protocol.*

Pocket Guide
to the Protocol

➢ The only time that you should pick a low-fat or non-fat option is with dairy. This is because with dairy the fat has not been replaced with sugar in order to make it non-fat or low-fat. For example, a yogurt labeled low-fat without stating low sugar probably has more sugar than a regular yogurt, which is not preferred.

➢ Also be aware that many, many recipes can be adapted to fit into maintenance with artificial sweeteners like Lakanto and stevia. There are countless resources for low carbohydrate/ sugar-free recipes, which should meet the criteria for maintenance phase.

➢ **To avoid a looming Steak Day**, as some participants do not necessarily care for a huge steak or not eating until the evening: drink lots of water throughout the day, don't eat until lunch, have a whole can of tuna (water packed) or chicken with mayo on **lettuce or celery for lunch**, have a big portion of protein for dinner with a small salad and 0-1 carbohydrate dressing (ex. Ranch). If you are extremely hungry, you could also have 2 eggs for breakfast. Note: This is not meant to take the place of a steak day (when you weight is more than 2 pounds over last HCG weight). This is used to drop some weight when you are getting close to a required Steak Day as it will usually bring your weight down a pound or so the next day.

Tasty Tips for the Maintenance Phase

➢ Maintenance Phase (P3) chocolate recipe: If you like strawberries or other fruit dipped in chocolate, heat 1Tbsp virgin coconut oil, 1½ Tbsp cocoa powder, and stevia to taste in a small sauce pan. Dip fruit and enjoy. Variation: Place chocolate on wax/parchment paper and freeze. You can also add a small amount of nuts or flavor extracts to make chocolate bark.

➢ Maintenance Phase (P3) chicken recipe: Mix ½ almond meal, ½ parmesan cheese. Bread your chicken breast with it and bake or pan fry in olive oil.

➢ Maintenance Phase (P3) Crustless Pumpkin Pie recipe: 15 minutes to prepare and cook.
  Ingredients:
    1 3/4 cup (1 small can) pumpkin
    2 eggs
    1 cup fat free milk
    2 tsp cinnamon
    1/2 tsp ginger
    1/2 tsp nutmeg
    1 cup no calorie sweetener (one that measures like sugar)
  Directions: Put all ingredients in a microwave safe bowl. Beat with a wire whisk to mix. Put in microwave uncovered. Cook on high for 8-10 minutes, depending on the power of your microwave, checking pie half way thru. Pie is done when the outside edges start to pull away from the sides just a little, and knife inserted in middle doesn't quite come out clean. Take out of microwave and cover bowl with a plate for about 5 minutes to finish cooking center. Cut into 6 pieces like you would a pie. Serve warm or cold. Makes 6 servings.

  Per serving: Calories: 62, Carbohydrates: 7g, Sugars: 4.3g, Protein: 4.6g, Fat: 1. g, Fiber: 3g (This took less than 15 minutes and was so easy and a really good substitute for the real deal, especially with a little real whip cream, also allowed on P3.) This is a nice holiday treat!

➢ Maintenance Phase (P3) Apple Pancake recipe for when you need a treat: finely chop 1 small apple, add ¼ tsp cinnamon, 2 packets stevia, and just enough pancake mix (mixed per the instructions) to coat the apple. Make like a regular pancake and serve with a little sugar-free syrup. If you only use 3 Tbsp of pancake batter, it would not constitute 'a starch'. Of course, this is a caution item, so don't overdo it.

Most Common Concerns during the Maintenance Phase (P3)

When people have a hard time on this phase it is usually due to one of three reasons:

1.) **Not eating enough food, especially protein** – most participants should eat a minimum of 1500 calories. In general, we do not encourage counting calories, but if you are a lifetime dieter, you may try to keep eating too little to avoid gaining back the weight you just lost. This is a major, common mistake. In these circumstances we encourage someone to add up the calories to make sure they are eating enough (not to limit what they are eating). According to Dr. Simeons, HCG is releasing 1500 to 4000 calories into your system and you are eating another 500 calories, so theoretically your system has been revved up to handle 2000 – 4500 calories PER DAY. You can see how going into the maintenance phase and 'cutting back' to 800 or 1200 would send your body back into the 'grab everything and hold on to it' / starvation mode.

2.) **Eating sugars and starches (intentionally or not)** – ex. Pizza is a starch! If you don't have a strong knowledge of food groups, refer to the "What can I eat and drink?" section of this book. The section lists many foods along with indicators for when the foods are allowed during the different phases of the HCG protocol. Keep in mind, most fruits are allowed, but use caution with both the starchy fruits like bananas/grapes and the super sweet ones like melons. The same applies for vegetables; most are allowed, but use caution with the starchy ones like Mexican beans, etc.

3.) **Staying on the 500 calorie diet a little too long** -- per Dr. Simeons:

> "When abnormal fat is no longer being put into circulation either because it has been consumed or because immunity has set in…,the body starts consuming normal fat, and this is always regained as soon as ordinary feeding is resumed. The patient then finds that the 2 - 3 lbs. he has lost during the last days of treatment are immediately regained. A meal is skipped and maybe a pound is lost. The next day this pound is regained, in spite of a careful watch over the food intake. In a few days a tearful patient is back in the consulting room, convinced that her case is a failure.

> All that is happening is that the essential fat lost at the end of the treatment, owing to the patient's reluctance to report a much greater hunger, is being replaced. The weight at which such a patient must stabilize thus lies 2 - 3 lbs. higher than the weight reached at the end of the treatment. Once this higher basic level is established, further difficulties in controlling the weight at the new point of stabilization hardly arise."

In this case, simply add 2 - 3 pounds to last HCG weight, and follow the normal guidelines for maintenance.

Maintenance Special Note:

We have seen a small percentage of participants (less than 3 %) who do everything right both during the diet phase and during the maintenance phase, but still somewhat "struggle" to maintain the weight loss. These people (including myself) have usually struggled their entire lives to keep weight gain to a minimum, but were basically always on a slight increase, with no hope of long term loss or maintenance. So, while this is not the ideal results for the protocol, some participants may have to simply pay more attention and stay more on guard to maintain their goal weight. For example, if a participant has been struggling, dieting and sacrificing, just to stay in a size 14, 16 or 20, they may still have to pay more attention than most participants to stay in their new size 8. The struggle is less after correctly performing the HCG protocol, but it still may exist to some degree. The good news is that slightly struggling in a size 8 is a lot more fun and a lot more comfortable than hopelessly struggling in a size 14 or 20.

Final Phase (Phase 4 as referenced in Trudeau's book)

As with Phase 1, Phase 4 in Kevin Trudeau's book is not directly from Dr. Simeons' manuscript. Again, it is more widely focused to include optimal health vs. purely weight loss/maintenance. After losing your excess weight, this wider focus is certainly appropriate. This is another reason we feel reading Trudeau's book after completing the HCG protocol is possibly more helpful than before beginning the protocol, as we feel before it is simply too overwhelming with the 100% organic food being demanded, along with many teas, cleanses and other 'products'.

If maintaining weight loss continues to be a struggle, I recommend purchasing the book and DVD, ***The Gabriel Method*** which may help address underlying issues that may be working against your weight loss success. Additionally, we have found the following guidelines to be simple, direct and effective in maintaining overall health:

- Take a multi-mineral / multi-vitamin daily
- Use a probiotic / digestive enzyme (preferably plant based) daily
- Include Amino Acids i.e. fish oil or flax seed oil daily
- Include live food i.e. uncooked, live fruit and or vegetables and natural organic protein (preferably not injected with hormones or antibiotics) at every meal.
- Drink lots of pure water
- Eat real food, like lean meats, fish, colored vegetables, fresh fruits, without chemical if possible.
- Eat healthy fats like almonds and coconut oil
- Get a good night's sleep (approximately 8 hours)
- Reduce stress
- Exercise a few times a week
- Do something you love
- Keep socializing with family and friends a priority

These tips may give you the edge that is needed to maintain your weight loss and eat like a normal, healthy person without fear of gaining the weight back.

Weight Chart for Women

Weight in pounds, based on ages 25-59 with the lowest mortality rate (indoor clothing weighing 3 pounds and shoes with 1" heels)

Height	Small Frame	Medium Frame	Large Frame
4'10"	102-111	109-121	118-131
4'11"	103-113	111-123	120-134
5'0"	104-115	113-126	122-137
5'1"	106-118	115-129	125-140
5'2"	108-121	118-132	128-143
5'3"	111-124	121-135	131-147
5'4"	114-127	124-138	134-151
5'5"	117-130	127-141	137-155
5'6"	120-133	130-144	140-159
5'7"	123-136	133-147	143-163
5'8"	126-139	136-150	146-167
5'9"	129-142	139-153	149-170
5'10"	132-145	142-156	152-173
5'11"	135-148	145-159	155-176
6'0"	138-151	148-162	158-179

Weight Chart for Men

Weight in pounds, based on ages 25-59 with the lowest mortality rate (indoor clothing weighing 5 pounds and shoes with 1" heels)

Height	Small Frame	Medium Frame	Large Frame
5'2"	128-134	131-141	138-150
5'3"	130-136	133-143	140-153
5'4"	132-138	135-145	142-156
5'5"	134-140	137-148h	144-160
5'6"	136-142	139-151	146-164
5'7"	138-145	142-154	149-168
5'8"	140-148	145-157	152-172
5'9"	142-151	148-160	155-176
5'10"	144-154	151-163	158-180
5'11"	146-157	154-166	161-184
6'0"	149-160	157-170	164-188
6'1"	152-164	160-174	168-192
6'2"	155-168	164-178	172-197
6'3"	158-172	167-182	176-202
6'4"	162-176	171-187	181-207

*Ideal Weights according to the Metropolitan Life Insurance Company tables

Calculating Your Frame Size

1. Extend your arm in front of your body bending your elbow at a ninety degree angle to your body so that your forearm is parallel to your body.

2. Keep your fingers straight and turn the inside of your wrist towards your body.

3. Place your thumb and index finger on the two prominent bones on either side of your elbow, then measure the distance between the bones with a tape measure or calipers.

4. Compare to the chart. The chart lists elbow measurements for a medium frame. If your elbow measurement for that particular height is less than the number of inches listed, you are a small frame. If your elbow measurement for that particular height is more than the number of inches listed, you are a large frame.

Elbow Measurements for Medium Frame			
Men	Elbow Measurement	Women	Elbow Measurement
5'2" - 5'3"	2-1/2" to 2-7/8"	4'10"-4'11"	2-1/4" to 2-1/2"
5'4" - 5'7"	2-5/8" to 2-7/8"	5'0" - 5'3"	2-1/4" to 2-1/2"
5'8" - 5'11"	2-3/4" to 3"	5'4" - 5'7"	2-3/8" to 2-5/8"
6'0" - 6'3"	2-3/4" to 3-1/8"	5/8" - 5'11"	2-3/8" to 2-5/8"

Tracking Your Progress Form

Name: _____

Date:											
Weight:											
Neck											
Right Arm											
Left Arm											
Upper Chest											
Chest											
Midriff											
Waist											
Hips											
Right Thigh											
Right Knee											
Right Calf											
Left Thigh											
Left Knee											
Left Calf											
Other (UR LR BB)											
Other											
Total Inches Lost											

Notes:
Neck - Standing, measure your neck at its largest girth, right over the Adam's apple

Arm – Armpit, then straight around

Upper Chest – at under arm level

Chest – At largest part

Midriff – directly under the bust line

Waist – Standing, measure at the narrowest point or at the midway point between the top of the hip bone and the bottom of the rib cage. If you can't find it, bend to the side and note where the bend is.

Hips - Measure at the largest girth, where the butt is protruding the greatest

Thigh – at largest part (top of the leg)

Knee – 1 inch above the top of the knee cap

Calf – at the largest part

Other (ex. Roll 1) – For example, if the belly button (BB) is not at the waist, note the BB. If there is a significant roll above the belly button (upper roll/UR) and / or below the belly button (lower roll/LR), you should note the measurements as these will change drastically and neither the waist or hip measurement will indicate the degree that these rolls change.

Instructions: The tape should be pulled to where it is lying flat against the skin all the way around. Your goal with body tape measurements is **consistency**. Take them the same every time you take them and you will get an accurate view of your progress with each body part.

Weight Loss Graph

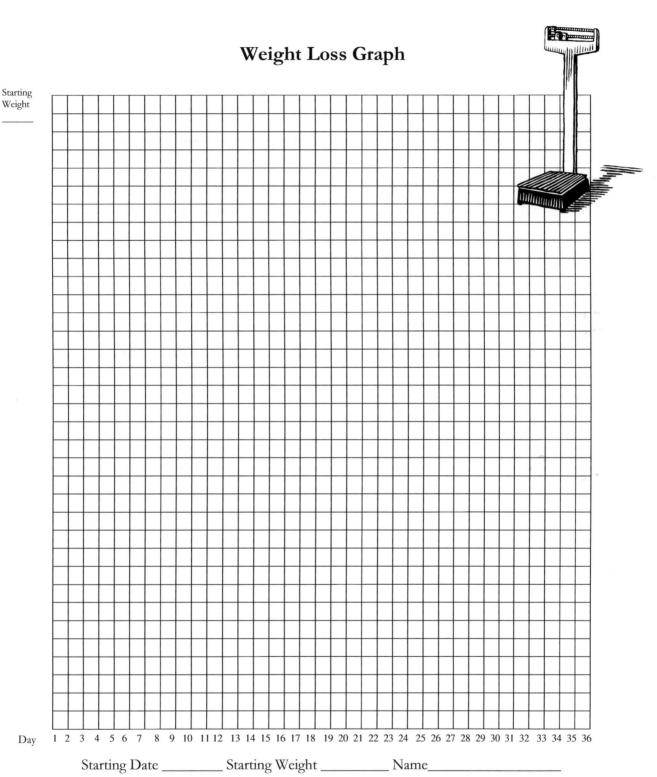

Starting
Weight
_____

Day 1 2 3 4 5 6 7 8 9 10 11 12 13 14 15 16 17 18 19 20 21 22 23 24 25 26 27 28 29 30 31 32 33 34 35 36

Starting Date _____ Starting Weight _____ Name_____

48

Daily Weight Log for All Phases of the HCG Protocol

Date	Weight	Any comments (how do you feel? good, tired, weak; if you cheated, etc.)	Date	Weight	Any comments (how do you feel? good, tired, weak; if you cheated, etc.)

What can I eat and drink?

Perhaps the most frequently asked question, once people actually start the HCG protocol, is **"What can I have on the 3 weeks No Sugar/No Starch phase?"**

The following list contains over 1000 food and beverage items and indicates which phase(s) allow each item. Some may disagree with some of the recommendations; after all, there isn't even agreement in the nutritional, government, and science communities about whether several foods are a fruit or a vegetable, i.e. cucumbers, tomatoes, pumpkins, to mention a few.

Interesting information on the fruits vs. vegetable quandary from U.S. Supreme Court in 1893
(Source: http://supreme.justia.com/us/149/304/case.html):

NIX v. HEDDEN, 149 U.S. 304 (1893)
Botanically speaking a tomato is the ovary, together with its seeds, of a flowering plant. This would mean that technically it would be considered a fruit. However, speaking from a culinary perspective the tomato is typically served as or part of a main course of a meal meaning that it would be considered a vegetable. This argument has lead to actual legal implications in the United States. In 1887, U.S. tariff laws which imposed a duty on vegetables but not on fruits caused the tomato's status to become a matter of legal importance. The U.S. Supreme Court settled this controversy in 1893, declaring that the tomato is a vegetable, along with cucumbers, squashes, beans, and peas, using the popular definition which classifies vegetables in how they are used: they are generally served with dinner and not dessert. The case is known as Nix v. Hedden

Some lists of vegetables have disclaimers stating, "Note that some herbs and vegetables which are botanically fruits are considered to be vegetables in the culinary sense."

Based on the above excerpt, botanically speaking, a pumpkin is a fruit, just as are tomatoes, cucumbers, squashes, avocados, green, yellow, and red peppers and peapods. Of course, we know Dr. Simeons did not go by this definition since tomatoes and cucumbers are both listed as vegetable choices on the 500 calorie diet phase. Consequently, we generally follow the U. S. Supreme Court's declaration: the tomato is a vegetable, along with cucumbers, squashes, beans, and peas, using the popular definition which classifies vegetables in how they are used and that they are generally served with dinner and not dessert.

There are also differences of opinion on exactly what Dr. Simeons meant for the first three weeks of maintenance when he said the following:

"During this period patients must realize that the so-called carbohydrate, that is sugar, rice, bread, potatoes, pastries etc, are by far the most dangerous. If no carbohydrates whatsoever are eaten, fats can be indulged in somewhat more liberally and even small quantities of alcohol, such as a glass of wine with meals, does no harm,…"

"Some patients cannot believe that they can eat fairly normally without regaining weight. They disregard the advice to eat anything they please except sugar and starch and want to play safe."

"For the following 3 weeks, all foods allowed except starch and sugar in any form (careful with very sweet fruit)."

Since small amounts of alcohol, such as a glass of wine with meals is described to do no harm, we contend that sugar and starch items are items that have a significant amount of carbohydrates and/or sugar, not items that have 4 grams or less, for example, of sugar in a serving. So while, cookies, cakes, candy, etc are clearly 'sugars', a teaspoon of ketchup on a hamburger does not constitute 'a sugar'. Nor do sweet fruits constitute a sugar, but they must be eaten with caution tempered by the daily weighing.

The same argument exists for starches. Dr. Simeons mentions items that are clearly considered 'starches', he gives no examples of vegetables that are starchy, such as beans or other vegetable that have protein and fiber. Therefore, we contend that some starchy vegetables (the ones with redeeming benefits of protein and fiber) are allowed in small quantities, with caution and these are all clearly marked.

There is a method to our madness, so if you disagree, you will know why an item was classified one way or another (more than 4 grams of sugar per serving counts as a 'sugar'; more than 13 grams of carbohydrate counts as a 'starch'), and you can decide for yourself how conservative you would like to proceed. If you want to stay extremely conservative, simply do not use any of the foods that are marked with the caution sign (Δ) until the food is no longer a caution food and your new weight is stabilized.

General food category information:
Fats contain 45 calories and 5 grams of fat per serving.
Fruits contain 15 grams of carbohydrate and 60 calories.
Lean Protein choices have 55 calories and 2-3 grams of fat per serving.
Medium Fat Proteins have 75 calories and 5 grams of fat per serving.
Starches contain 15 grams of carbohydrate and 80 calories per serving.
Vegetables contain about 25 calories and about 5 grams of carbohydrate.

Fruit: An apple has 19 carbohydrates, 3 fibers, and 14 sugar grams. Since apples are allowed on all phases and Dr. Simeons only suggests caution with 'very sweet' fruit. Therefore, if a fruit has 14 or more grams of sugar per serving with less than 3 fibers or with more than 20 carbohydrates, the fruit is classified as caution (Δ).

Vegetables: Generally, vegetables contain about 25 calories and about 5 grams of carbohydrate. If a vegetable has less than 10 grams of carbohydrates, the vegetable is classified as free to eat in the maintenance phase. If a vegetable has 10 – 13 grams of fiber without protein and/or fiber, the vegetable is considered a starchy vegetable and is classified as caution (Δ) for maintenance. If a vegetable has more than 13 fibers without significant protein and/or fiber, the vegetable is considered a starch. Beans and legumes are some of the vegetables that contain more calories and more carbohydrates, but many also include significant protein and fiber. For these reasons, several earn the classification of caution (Δ) for the maintenance phase as many people have no problem having limited portions due to the high protein/fiber combination. On the other hand, if these have 3 or grams of sugar, you may be best advised to avoid for the first three weeks of maintenance or extreme caution (Δ)* is advised. Different brands vary in nutritional content for most items, so a quick reference on any can or package is advisable.

Other notes: While in general this book recommends eating real food in full form vs. light, fat-free or sugar-free, dairy products are the exception. Low fat and non fat dairy products such as cheese, milk, yogurt are considered healthy alternatives because the products are skimmed after the fat rises to the top during processing and nothing is generally added to make up for that fat. However, the other low fat and non fat items such as crackers, cereal, mayonnaise, salad dressing, etc, are not recommended as the added carbohydrates replace fat with sugar and carbohydrates.

Most of the information used to compile the food item, Serving Size, Calories, Protein (Pro), Carbohydrate (Carb), Fiber, Sugar, Fat, and Saturated Fat (Sat Fat) columns **ONLY** are from The Biggest Loser Complete Calorie Counter copyrighted in 2006, which sources included the ESHA Research Food Processor program, manufacturers' Web site, restaurant submissions and Web sites, and the USDA National Nutrient Database for Standard Reference – Release 18. Other sources such as nutrition labels directly off cans and the Web sites listed below were also sources for the information. If specific nutrients were not listed, the columns have n/a listed.

The other four columns displayed below are based on our research, opinion and guidelines as stated above.

500 Diet	1st 3 wks	2nd 3 wks	Life

These columns indicate which phases (500 calorie diet phase, 1st 3 weeks of maintenance phase, 2nd 3 weeks of maintenance phase, and the rest of your life) each of these items are considered allowable. Many HCG protocol participants have followed these guidelines with notable success through all phases.

General Outline of Beverage/Food Items

Beverages
    Alcohol
    Coffee, Hot Chocolate and Tea
    Juice
    Milk and Non Dairy
    Other Drink
Entrees
    Eggs
    Fish
    Meat
        Alligator
        Beef
        Bison
        Boar
        Chicken
        Duck
        Lamb
        Pork
        Veal
        Turkey
        Seafood
        Other (Breakfast
        Burrito/Sandwich, Beef Stew,
        Chicken/Tuna Salad, Chili,
        Pizza, Quiche, Soup
Fruit
Vegetable
Nut, Nut Butter and Seeds
Dairy Products
    Cheese
    Cream
    Whipped Topping
    Yogurt

Starches
    Bread
    Crackers
    Cereal
    Flour
    Grains and Rice
Desserts & Sweet Treats
    Candy
    Baked goods
    Frozen yogurt
    Ice cream
    Ice cream topping
Snacks
    Baked chips
    Jerky
    Popcorn
    Pork skins
    Potato chips
    Pretzels
    Rice cakes
    Trail mix
    Wasabi peas
Condiments
Fats & Oils
Sweeteners
    Artificial
    Natural
Herbs & Spices
Sauces & Gravy

In the following list of items, the symbols N, Y, Δ, and Δ* are used to indicate whether or not each item listed is allowed during each phase of the HCG protocols:

N = No, this item is not allowed during this phase of the protocol.

Y = Yes, this item should be fine, unless taken to an extreme.

Δ = Caution, both in quantity and frequency, should be used. Also, don't combine too many 'cautions' in one day.

Δ* = Extreme Caution: If you want to be conservative, you may want to avoid these items during this phase usually due to the small amount of sugar that may or may not be listed on the nutritional information, but probably included in the ingredients list.

Some of the sources used for nutritional information in the following food list:

The Biggest Loser Complete Calorie Counter

http://low-carb.com/natalflour16.html

http://www24.netrition.com/simply_coconut_flour_page.html

http://www.bluediamond.com/retail/breeze/Almond

You can use the following websites to find nutritional information on almost anything:

http://www.fns.usda.gov/

http://www.calorieking.com/

http://www.nal.usda.gov/fnic/foodcomp/search/

A good source for fast food restaurant foods: http://www.dietfacts.com/fastfood.asp

Beverages

Food/Item	Serving Size	Calories	Pro	Carb	Fiber	Sugar	Fat	Sat Fat	500 Diet	1st 3 wks	2nd 3 wks	Life
Alcohol												
aquavit, bourbon, brandy, gin, rum, tequila, vodka, whiskey, 86 proof	1.5 oz	104	0	0	0	0	0	0	N	Δ	Δ	Y
beer, regular	12 oz	150	1	13	n/a	n/a	0	0	N	N	Δ	Y
black Russian cocktail	1.5 oz	115	0	8	0	6	0	0	N	N	Δ	Y
Bloody Mary	8 oz	50	1	8	1	5	0	0	N	N	Δ	Y
coffee and cream liqueur	1.5 oz	153	1	10	0	9	7	5	N	N	Δ	Y
coffee liqueur, 63 proof	1.5 oz	161	0	17	0	17	0	0	N	N	Δ	Y
daiquiri	8 oz	185	0	47	1	46	0	0	N	N	Δ	Y
gin and tonic cocktail	6 oz	117	0	6	0	6	0	0	N	N	Δ	Y
Harvey Wallbanger	6 oz	145	1	15	0	15	0	0	N	N	Δ	Y
margarita	1.5 oz	94	0	6	0	6	0	0	N	N	Δ	Y
martini	1.5 oz	103	0	1	0	0	0	0	N	Δ	Δ	Y
pina colada	1.5 oz	82	0	11	0	n/a	1	1	N	N	Δ	Y
sangria	5 oz	98	0	13	0	n/a	0	0	N	N	Δ	Y
screwdriver	6 oz	145	1	15	0	15	0	0	N	N	Δ	Y
sloe gin fizz	6 oz	93	0	2	0	n/a	0	0	N	Δ	Δ	Y
whiskey sour cocktail	6 oz	289	0	28	0	28	0	0	N	N	Δ	Y
white Russian	1.5 oz	109	0	7	0	6	1	0	N	N	Δ	Y
wine cooler or spritzer	5 oz	59 - 71	0	1-8	0	n/a	0	0	N	Δ	Δ	Y
wine: dry burgundy, cabernet claret, red, sherry, white (Chenin Blanc, Gewurztraminer, medium, Pinot Grigio, Sauvignon, Semillon)	5 oz	102 - 131	0	2-5.5	n/a	2-5.5	0	0	N	Δ	Δ	Y

Food/Item	Serving Size	Calories	Pro	Carb	Fiber	Sugar	Fat	Sat Fat	500 Diet	1st 3 wks	2nd 3 wks	Life
wine: dessert (dry or sweet) , Japanese rice, Marsala, plum, port, rice (sake), white (vermouth)	5 oz	195 - 236	0	~ 23	0	~ 23	0	n/a	N	N	Δ	Y
wine: mirin	5 oz	336	1	47	0	47	0	0	N	N	Δ	Δ

Coffee, Hot Chocolate and Tea Items

cappuccino, fat free milk	8 oz	53	5	7	0	7	0	0	N	Δ	Y	Y
cappuccino, low-fat milk	8 oz	73	5	7	0	7	2	2	N	Δ	Y	Y
coffee, brewed or instant, regular or decaf	8 oz	0 - 12	0-1	0-2	0	0	0	0	Y	Y	Y	Y
coffee, latte -single or double w/fat-free milk	8 oz	47	5	7	0	6	0	0	N	Δ	Y	Y
coffee, latte -single or double, w/ low-fat milk	8 oz	60	5	7	0	6	2	1	N	Δ	Y	Y
coffee, latte, with Silk soy, regular or spicy	8 oz	145-170	5-6	20-29	0	18-23	4	0	N	N	Δ	Y
coffee, mocha, with fat-free milk	8 oz	120	8	22	1	19	1	0	N	N	Δ	Y
coffee, mocha, with low-fat milk	8 oz	200	8	22	1	19	10	6	N	N	Δ	Y
espresso, regular or decaf	4 oz	11	0	2	0	2	0	0	Y	Y	Y	Y
tea: regular or decaf black, chamomile, herbal, mint	8 oz	0 - 2	0	0	0	0	0	0	Y	Y	Y	Y
hot cocoa, sugar-free, with water	8 oz	66	3	12	1	0	1	0	N	Δ	Y	Y
hot cocoa, sugar-free, with low-fat milk	8 oz	158	8	27	1	n/a	3	2	N	N	Y	Y
hot cocoa, with water	8 oz	125	2	26	1	23	1	1	N	N	Δ	Y
hot cocoa, with whole milk	8 oz	193	7	27	1	n/a	8	5	N	N	Δ	Y

Juice

Aloe Vera juice	4 oz	45	1	11	0	0	0	0	N	Δ	Y	Y
apple juice	4 oz	58	0	14	0	14	0	0	N	N	Y	Y
carrot juice	4 oz	47	1	11	1	5	0	0	N	Δ	Δ	Y
cherry juice	4 oz	70	0	17	0	16	0	0	N	N	Δ	Y
cranberry juice	4 oz	58	0	15	0	15	0	0	N	N	Δ	Y
grape juice	4 oz	77	1	19	0	19	0	0	N	N	Δ	Y
grapefruit juice	4 oz	47	1	11	0	11	0	0	N	Δ	Δ	Y
guava juice drink	4 oz	66	0	17	1	16	0	0	N	N	Δ	Y
lemon juice	4 oz	30	0	10	0	3	0	0	N	Y	Y	Y
lime juice	4 oz	31	1	10	0	2	0	0	N	Y	Y	Y
mango nectar juice	4 oz	72	0	19	1	18	0	0	N	N	Δ	Y
orange juice	4 oz	56	1	13	0	10	0	0	N	Δ	Y	Y
passion fruit juice	4 oz	63	0	17	0	17	0	0	N	N	Δ	Y
pineapple juice	4 oz	66	0	16	0	12	0	0	N	N	Δ	Y
pomegranate juice	4 oz	70	1	18	0	17	0	0	N	N	Δ	Y
prune juice	4 oz	90	1	22	1	21	0	0	N	N	Δ	Y
tomato juice	4 oz	21	1	5	0	4	0	0	N	Y	Y	Y
vegetable juice V8	4 oz	25	1	5	1	4	0	0	N	Y	Y	Y

Milk and Nondairy

almond,												
original	8 oz	60	1	8	1	7	2.5	0	N	Δ	Y	Y
original, unsweetened	8 oz	40	1	2	1	0	3	0	N	Δ	Y	Y

Food/Item	Serving Size	Calories	Pro	Carb	Fiber	Sugar	Fat	Sat Fat	500 Diet	1st 3 wks	2nd 3 wks	Life
Milk and Nondairy (cont)												
chocolate	8 oz	120	2	22	1	20	3	0	N	N	Δ	Y
chocolate, unsweetened	8 oz	45	2	3	1	0	3.5	0	N	Δ	Y	Y
vanilla	8 oz	90	1	16	1	15	2.5	0	N	N	Δ	Y
vanilla, unsweetened	8 oz	40	1	2	1	0	3	0	N	Δ	Y	Y
buttermilk, cultured, low-fat	1 oz	110	10	14	0	14	2	1	N	N	Δ	Y
evaporated milk, fat-free	4 oz	88	7	14	0	14	0	0	N	N	Δ	Y
half-and-half	1 oz	37	1	1	0	1	0	0	N	Δ	Y	Y
hot cocoa, sugar-free, with water	8 oz	66	3	12	1	0	1	0	N	Δ	Y	Y
hot cocoa, sugar-free, with low-fat milk	8 oz	158	8	27	1	n/a	3	2	N	N	Y	Y
hot cocoa, with water	8 oz	125	2	26	1	23	1	1	N	N	Δ	Y
hot cocoa, with whole milk	8 oz	193	7	27	1	n/a	8	5	N	N	Δ	Y
milk, fat-free	1 c	90	9	13	0	12	0	0	N	Δ	Y	Y
milk, low-fat 1%	1 c	118	10	14	0	11	3	2	N	Δ	Y	Y
milk, reduced-fat 2%	1 c	122	8	11	0	11	5	3	N	Δ	Y	Y
milk, whole	1 c	146	8	11	0	11	8	5	N	Δ	Δ	Y
rice milk	1 c	144	3	28	2	n/a	2	0	N	N	Δ	Y
soy milk	1 c	127	11	12	3	1	5	1	N	Δ	Y	Y
soy milk, light	1 c	70	6	8	1	6	2	0	N	Δ	Y	Y

Food/Item	Serving Size	Calories	Pro	Carb	Fiber	Sugar	Fat	Sat Fat	500 Diet	1st 3 wks	2nd 3 wks	Life
Other Drinks												
Bottled water: plain, 0 Water (all flavors), Perrier	8 oz	0	0	0	0	0	0	0	Y	Y	Y	Y
club soda, also known as carbonated water, soda water, sparkling water, fizzy water, club soda, or seltzer water	8 oz	0	0	0	0	0	0	0	N	Y	Y	Y
Fresca Sparkling drinks: Black Cherry, Peach	8 oz	20	0	5	n/a	5	0	n/a	N	Y	Y	Y
Glaceau Fruit Water: grape, lime, peach, raspberry	8 oz	20	0	5	n/a	5	0	n/a	N	Y	Y	Y
soda												
cola, regular	8 oz	100	0	25.5	0	25.5	0	0	N	N	Δ	Y
cola, diet	8 oz	0-1	0	0	0	0	0	0	N	Y	Y	Y
Crystal Light, any flavor	1 serving	5	0	0	n/a	0	0	n/a	N	Y	Y	Y
Snapple, diet, all flavors	8 oz	0-10	0	1-4	n/a	0-3	0	n/a	N	Y	Y	Y

Entrees
Eggs, Fish, Meat, Seafood,
Other Miscellaneous

Food/Item	Serving Size	Calories	Pro	Carb	Fiber	Sugar	Fat	Sat Fat	500 Diet	1st 3 wks	2nd 3 wks	Life
Eggs												
egg	1 large	74-78	6	0	0	0	5	2	Δ	Y	Y	Y
egg white, raw	1 large	17	4	0	0	0	0	0	Δ	Y	Y	Y

Fish												
caviar: red or black	1 tbsp	40	4	1	0	0	3	1	N	Δ	Y	Y
Low fat, low calorie and allowed during 500 calorie phase: bass, sea or striped, burbot, cisco, Atlantic cod, Pacific cod, cusk, dolphin*, mahi-mahi*, flounder, grouper, haddock, ling, ling cod, mahi-mahi*, monkfish, northern pike, ocean perch (Atlantic), orange roughy, pike (walleye), pollock (Atlantic), rockfish (Pacific), rainbow smelt, snapper, sole, tarpon*, tilapia, walleye pike, whiting, wolffish (Atlantic), raw *These items meet the nutritional criteria of other 500 calorie phase fish and are not specifically excluded by Dr. Simeons, but some might consider these questionable. If you want to be conservative, you may wish to avoid for this phase.	4 oz	81-109					1-2		Y	Y	Y	Y
Low fat, low calorie, but not allowed during 500 calorie phase: carp, brown trout, catfish (wild or farmed), cisco, croaker, devilish (Alaskan), dolphin*, drumfish, halibut (Atlantic) mackerel (king), mahi-mahi*, mullet (striped), salmon (chum, pink), scallops*, shark, smelt (rainbow), snapper, sturgeon, swordfish, trout (wild, rainbow), tarpon*, tilefish, trout (sea), tuna (slipjack, yellowfin), tuna (white, canned in water), turbot, whitefish (Atlantic) wolffish (Atlantic), raw	4 oz	108-153	13-27	0-1	0	0	2-9	0-1	N	Y	Y	Y
More (high) fat and calories: butterfish, herring, Greenland halibut, mackerel (Atlantic, Pacific, Spanish), milkfish, sablefish, salmon (Atlantic, chinock, Coho, sockeye), shad, tuna (bluefin), raw	4 oz	158-240	15-24	0	0	0	2-9	2-4	N	Y	Y	Y

Meat												
alligator	3 oz	197	39	0	0	0	4	0	N	Y	Y	Y
beef												
bottom round, cooked	3 oz	139	24	0	0	0	5	2	Y	Y	Y	Y
brisket flat, lean	3 oz	174	28	0	0	0	6	2	N	Y	Y	Y

Food/Item	Serving Size	Calories	Pro	Carb	Fiber	Sugar	Fat	Sat Fat	500 Diet	1st 3 wks	2nd 3 wks	Life
Entrees: Meat, Beef (cont)												
chuck roast, lean	3 oz	179	28	0	0	0	6	2	N	Y	Y	Y
corned beef, cooked	3 oz	215	15	0	0	0	16	5	N	Y	Y	Y
cotto salami, beef	1 oz	58	4	1	0	0	4	2	N	Y	Y	Y
eye round, lean cooked	3 oz	138	25	0	0	0	3	1	Y	Y	Y	Y
filet mignon, lean, broiled	3 oz	179	24	0	0	0	9	3	Δ	Y	Y	Y
flank steak, lean broiled	3 oz	158	24	0	0	0	6	3	Y	Y	Y	Y
ground beef, 80% lean, broiled	3 oz	230	22	0	0	0	15	6	N	Y	Y	Y
ground beef, extra lean, raw	4 oz	130	22	0	0	0	5	2	Δ	Y	Y	Y
hot dog, beef, 97% fat free	1.7 oz	45	6	3	0	0	1	1	N	Δ	Y	Y
jerky, beef	1 oz	116	9.5	3.1	.5	2.6	7.3	3.1	N	Δ	Y	Y
rib pot roast, lean, roasted	3 oz	131	15	0	0	0	7	3	Y	Y	Y	Y
rib steak, lean, roasted	3 oz	81	11	0	0	0	4	2	Y	Y	Y	Y
roast, lean, roasted	3 oz	169	24	0	0	0	7	3	Δ	Y	Y	Y
roast beef, lunch meat	1 oz	30-35	6-7	1	0	0	4	2	N	Y	Y	Y
salami, beef, cooked	1 oz	73	4	1	0	0	6	2	N	Y	Y	Y
salami, beef, lean, sliced	1 oz	45	4	1	0	0	2	1	N	Y	Y	Y
short ribs, lean, w/bone, braised	3 oz	65	7	0	0	0	4	2	N	Y	Y	Y
sirloin steak, broiled	3 oz	236	22	0	0	0	16	6	N	Y	Y	Y
top sirloin steak, lean, broiled	3 oz	166	26	0	0	0	6	2	Δ	Y	Y	Y
stew meat, lean, cooked	3 oz	201	27	0	0	0	10	4	N	Y	Y	Y
t-bone, lean, broiled	3 oz	168	22	0	0	0	8	3	Δ	Y	Y	Y
tenderloin, lean, boneless	4 oz	163	24	0	0	0	6	2	Δ	Y	Y	Y
top round steak, braised	3 oz	177	24	0	0	0	8	3	Δ	Y	Y	Y
bison												
bison, ground, pan broiled	3 oz	202	20	0	0	0	13	6	Δ	Y	Y	Y
bison, roast, roasted	3 oz	123	24	0	0	0	2	1	Y	Y	Y	Y
boar, wild, cooked	3 oz	136	24	0	0	0	4	1	N	Y	Y	Y
chicken												
buffalo wing, spicy	3 oz	261	22	0	0	0	19	5	N	Y	Y	Y
chicken, breast, without skin, cooked	3 oz	128	25	0	0	0	3	1	Y	Y	Y	Y
chicken, breast, fat-free sliced	3 oz	67	14	2	0	0	0	0	Y	Y	Y	Y
chicken, drumstick/thigh, cooked	3 oz	149-174	15-22	0	0	0	5-9	1-2	N	Y	Y	Y
hot dog, chicken	1	116	6	3	0	0	9	2	N	Δ	Y	Y
chicken liver pate	1 oz	57	4	2	0	0	4	1	N	Y	Y	Y
chicken lunch meat, deli	1 oz	30	6	1	0	1	1	0	N	Y	Y	Y
duck												
duck, breast, without skin	3 oz	119	23	0	0	0	2	0	N	Y	Y	Y
duck, whole, roasted, chopped	3 oz	238-287	16-20	0	0	0	17-24	6-8	N	Y	Y	Y
emu: fan filet or ground, broiled	3 oz	131-139	24-27	0	0	0	2-4	1	N	Y	Y	Y
goose, whole, roasted	3 oz	259	21	0	0	0	18	6	N	Y	Y	Y
goat, baked, broiled, or roasted	3 oz	122	12	0	0	0	3	1	N	Y	Y	Y
lamb												
center slice, loin, ribs, sirloin chop	3 oz	160-183	21-23	0	0	0	7-10	3-6	N	Y	Y	Y
ground, broiled	3 oz	241	21	0	0	0	17	7	N	Y	Y	Y
ostrich: ground, top loin, cooked	3 oz	121-132	22-25	0	0	0	3-6	1-2	N	Y	Y	Y

Food/Item	Serving Size	Calories	Pro	Carb	Fiber	Sugar	Fat	Sat Fat	500 Diet	1st 3 wks	2nd 3 wks	Life
Entrees: Meat, (cont)												
pheasant, whole, cooked	3 oz	210	28	0	0	0	10	1	N	Y	Y	Y
pork												
bacon, cooked	.2 oz	34	2	0	0	0	3	1	N	Y	Y	Y
Canadian bacon, grilled	1 oz	52	7	0	0	0	2	1	N	Y	Y	Y
chitlins, cooked	1 oz	66	4	0	0	0	6	3	N	Y	Y	Y
chop, center lean w/bone, braised	2.6 oz	149	22	0	0	0	6	2	N	Y	Y	Y
chop sirloin, lean w/bone braised	2.5 oz	142	19	0	0	0	6	2	N	Y	Y	Y
ground, cooked	3 oz	253	22	0	0	0	18	7	N	Y	Y	Y
hot dog, pork	2.7 oz	204	10	0	0	0	18	7	N	Y	Y	Y
hot dog, pork, beef, and turkey, fat-free	1.8 oz	50	6	6	0	2	0	0	N	Δ	Y	Y
prosciutto, sliced	.5 oz	50	4	0	0	0	2	1	N	Y	Y	Y
pulled, with sauce	3 oz	147	13	8	0	n/a	7	2	N	Δ	Y	Y
ribs, country-style, lean, braised	3 oz	199	22	0	0	0	12	4	N	Y	Y	Y
roast, center loin, roasted	3 oz	169	23	0	0	0	8	3	N	Y	Y	Y
quail, whole, cooked	3 oz	199	21	0	0	0	12	3	N	Y	Y	Y
salami, Italian port	1 oz	120	6	0	0	0	10	4	N	Y	Y	Y
sausage, cooked	.5 oz	44	3	0	0	0	4	1	N	Y	Y	Y
scrapple	2 oz	119	5	8	0	0	8	3	N	Y	Y	Y
tenderloin, roasted	3 oz	139	24	0	0	0	4	1	N	Y	Y	Y
veal												
breast, braised	3 oz	226	23	0	0	0	14	6	N	Y	Y	Y
cube steak	3 oz	220	14	0	0	0	18	8	N	Y	Y	Y
ground, 8% fat, broiled	3 oz	146	21	0	0	0	6	3	Y	Y	Y	Y
leg, lean, cubed, braised	3 oz	160	30	0	0	0	4	1	Δ	Y	Y	Y
leg, top round steak, lean, roasted	3 oz	128	24	0	0	0	3	1	Y	Y	Y	Y
loin or loin chop, braised	3 oz	185-192	21-29	0	0	0	6-8	2	N	Y	Y	Y
loin chop cutlet, braised	3 oz	242	26	0	0	0	15	6	N	Y	Y	Y
shank roast, braised	3 oz	151	27	0	0	0	4	1	Y	Y	Y	Y
short rib, lean, roasted	3 oz	143	21	0	0	0	6	2	Y	Y	Y	Y
shoulder arm steak or blade roast, braised	3 oz	168-171	28-30	0	0	0	5-6	1-2	N	Y	Y	Y
sirloin roast or top round steak, lean, raw	4 oz	121-127	16-24	0	0	0	2-4	1	N	Y	Y	Y
turkey												
breast, roasted	3 oz	161	24	0	0	0	6	2	N	Y	Y	Y
dark meat, roasted	3 oz	159 – 188	23-24	0	0	0	5-10	2	N	Y	Y	Y
giblets, raw	1	315	47	5	0	0	10	3	N	Y	Y	Y
gizzard, raw	1	139	22	0	0	0	5	1	N	Y	Y	Y
ground, 11% fat, sausage	3 oz	146	14	0	0	0	10	3	N	Y	Y	Y
heart, raw	1	34	5	0	0	0	1	0	N	Y	Y	Y
leg, with skin, roasted	3 oz	177	24	0	0	0	8	3	N	Y	Y	Y
neck, without skin, raw	1	243	36	0	0	0	10	3	N	Y	Y	Y
hotdog, turkey	1	102	6	1	0	0	8	3	N	Y	Y	Y
jerky	1 oz	71-81	14	3-4	0	3-4	1	0	N	Δ	Y	Y
venison												
chop, cooked	3 oz	177	25	0	0	0	8	2	N	Y	Y	Y
stewed	3 oz	145	28	0	0	0	3	1	N	Y	Y	Y
jerky	1 oz	116	9.4	3.1	.5	2.6	7.3	3.1	N	Δ	Y	Y

Food/Item	Serving Size	Calories	Pro	Carb	Fiber	Sugar	Fat	Sat Fat	500 Diet	1st 3 wks	2nd 3 wks	Life
Seafood												
crab: Alaskan king, blue, Dungeness, queen, snow, steamed or baked	3 oz	83 – 117	16-20	0-1	0	0-1	0-2	0-1	Y	Y	Y	Y
crab cake	1	160	11	5	0	0	10	2	N	N	Δ	Y
crayfish, wild or farmed, steamed	3 oz	70-74	14-15	0	0	0	1	0	Y	Y	Y	Y
lobster, steamed	3 oz	83	17	1	0	0	1	0	Y	Y	Y	Y
scallops, raw	4 oz	100	18	3	0	0	1	0	Δ	Y	Y	Y
shrimp, cooked	3 oz	101	21	0	0	0	2	0	Y	Y	Y	Y
Other Main Entrees: soup, pizza, misc entrees												
beef stew	1 c	170	10	18	4	2	7	2	N	Δ	Δ	Y
breakfast burrito, ham and cheese	4 oz	210	9	30	0	2	6	2	N	N	Δ	Y
breakfast sandwich, bacon, egg, & cheese biscuit	1	441	20	33	1	3	27	7	N	N	Δ	Y
chicken salad	1/2 c	250	10	9	2	4	20	4	N	Δ	Y	Y
chili, without noodles, with beans and meat	1 c	203-287	15-19	26-30	6-11	3-6	3-14	0-6	N		Δ	Y
pizza												
cheese	1 slice	304	13	38	2	6	11	5	N	N	Δ	Y
pepperoni	1 slice	413	18	39	n/a	n/a	21	8	N	N	Δ	Y
sausage	1 slice	337	12	32	n/a	n/a	18	6	N	N	Δ	Y
vegetarian	1 slice	260	13	36	2	5	8	3	N	N	Δ	Y
quiche	1/8 pie	336	10	16	0	n/a	26	13	N	N	Δ	Y
Soup												
broth: beef or chicken	15-17	15 -17	1-3	0	0	0	1	0	Y	Y	Y	Y
soup, homemade: soup w/broth, with allowed protein, 1 allowed vegetable and allowed seasonings	1 c	75-150	17-25	0-7	0-3	0	0-5	0-3	Y	Y	Y	Y
soup, homemade: soup w/broth and/or cream, with allowed protein, most vegetables (except no starches of potatoes, corn, rice, etc.) and seasonings	1 c	n/a	n/a	0-13	n/a	< 2	n/a	n/a	N	Y	Y	Y
soup, homemade: soup w/potatoes, corn, noodles, rice or other foods not allowed on 500 calorie phase	1 c	n/a	n/a	>13	n/a	n/a	n/a	n/a	N	N	Δ	Y
soup, store bought: In general, you must read the label--if carbs are <13 and sugar < 2g i.e. beef and onion, cauliflower	1 c	n/a	n/a	0-13	n/a	<2	n/a	n/a	N	Y	Y	Y
soup, store bought: In general, you must read the label--if carbs are > 12 and/or sugars are 2 g or more, make sure un-allowed foods such as rice, noodles, potatoes, corn, etc. are **not** included	1 c	n/a	n/a	>14	n/a	< 4	n/a	n/a	N	Δ	Y	Y

Food/Item	Serving Size	Calories	Pro	Carb	Fiber	Sugar	Fat	Sat Fat	500 Diet	1st 3 wks	2nd 3 wks	Life
Other Entrees: soup, (cont)												
soup, store bought: In general, you must read the label-- if soup includes sugars and/or starches not allowed in the 1st 3 weeks, i.e. chicken rice or noodle, corn chowder, beef stroganoff	1 c	n/a	n/a	>19	n/a	>3	n/a	n/a	N	N	Δ	Y
soup, store bought samples (brands differ):												
beef/chicken and country vegetables	1 c	143	12	15	n/a	n/a	4	1	N	N	Δ	Y
beef /chicken/turkey mushroom	1 c	31	2	2.6	0	0	1.2	.6	N	Y	Y	Y
beef/chicken/turkey noodle	1 c	28 - 34	2	4-6	0-1	0	1	0	N	Y	Y	Y
beef stroganoff	1 c	173	9	16	2	2	9	3	N	N	Δ	Y
beef vegetable	1 c	32	2	4	0	0	1	0	N	Y	Y	Y
black bean	1/2 c	90	5	13	8	2	2	1	N	Δ	Y	Y
black bean, low-fat (notice more sugar)	1/2 c	70	4	13	3	4	1	0	N	N	Δ	Y
borscht	1 c	78	3	8	2	n/a	4	2	N	Δ	Y	Y
broccoli-cheese	1 c	180	6	12	n/a	n/a	12	4	N	Δ	Y	Y
chicken and wild rice	1 c	190	6	17	2	3	11	5	N	N	Δ	Y
chicken corn or mushroom chowder	1 c	192 - 225	7	17	2-3	n/a	11- 14	3-4	N	N	Δ	Y
chicken vegetable	1 c	70	3	8	1	1	2	1	N	Y	Y	Y
chicken vegetable, low-sodium - note significant differences	1 c	166	12	19	1	2	5	1	N	N	Δ	Y
clam chowder, Manhattan	1 c	78	2	12	1	1	2	0	N	Δ	Y	Y
clam chowder, New England	1 c	190	6	20	1	3	10	3	N	N	Δ	Y
clam chowder, New England, reduced fat	1 c	110	6	19	2	2	2	1	N	N	Δ	Y
crab	1 c	76	5	10	1	n/a	2	0	N	Δ	Y	Y
crab bisque	1 c	260	22	12	2	2	10	2	N	N	Δ	Y
cream of celery, 98% fat-free	1 c	120	2	16	2	2	6	2	N	N	Δ	Y
cream of tomato	1 c	130	3	26	2	18	2	1	N	N	Δ	Y
escarole	1 c	25	1	3	1	1	1	0	N	Δ	Y	Y
French onion	1 c	43	2	6	1	4	1	0	N	Δ	Y	Y
gazpacho	1 c	43	7	4	0	2	0	0	N	Δ	Y	Y
green pea	1 c	165	9	27	5	8	3	1	N	N	Y	Y
lentil	1 c	150	8	19	9	3	5	1	N	Δ	Y	Y
lobster bisque	1 c	400	3	11	0	4	39	24	N	N	Δ	Y
lobster gumbo	1 c	178	10	20	3	0	7	1.5	N	Δ	Y	Y
minestrone	1 c	120	5	22	4	4	2	0	N	N	Δ	Y
mushroom	1 c	96	2	11	1	0	5	1	N	Y	Y	Y
oyster stew	1 c	135	6	10	0	n/a	8	5	N	Y	Y	Y
potato	1 c	60	2	7	0	0	3	2	N	N	Δ	Y
ramen	1 package	140	8	26	4	4	1	0	N	N	Δ	Y
shrimp gumbo	1 c	158	10	18	2	n/a	6	2	N	Δ	Y	Y
split pea	1 c	100	7	19	4	4	0	0	N	Δ	Y	Y

Food/Item	Serving Size	Calories	Pro	Carb	Fiber	Sugar	Fat	Sat Fat	500 Diet	1st 3 wks	2nd 3 wks	Life
Other Entrees: soup, (cont)												
sweet and sour	1 c	72	3	14	2	n/a	1	0	N	Δ	Y	Y
tomato	1 c	161	6	22	3	15	6	3	N	N	Δ	Y
tomato bisque	1 c	179	6	27	0	n/a	6	3	N	N	Δ	Y
tomato garden	1 c	51	2	9	2	3	1	0	N	Δ	Y	Y
vegetable	1 c	70	3	8	1	1	3	1	N	Y	Y	Y
vegetable beef, chicken	1 c	50 -78	3-6	8-10	0	1	2	1	N	Y	Y	Y
tuna salad	1/2 c	260	12	9	2	4	19	3	N	Δ	Y	Y

Fruit

Food/Item	Serving Size	Calories	Pro	Carb	Fiber	Sugar	Fat	Sat Fat	500 Diet	1st 3 wks	2nd 3 wks	Life
apricot	1	17	0	4	1	3	0	0	N	Y	Y	Y
apple	1	72	0	19	3	14	0	0	Y	Y	Y	Y
apple, crab	1/2c	42	0	11	1	n/a	0	0	N	Y	Y	Y
applesauce, unsweetened	1/3 c	33	0	9	1	7	0	0	N	Y	Y	Y
applesauce, sweetened	1/3 c	64	0	17	1	14	0	0	N	Δ	Δ	Y
avocado	1/4 c	58	1	3	2	0	5	1	N	Y	Y	Y
banana	1 7"	105	1	27	3	14	0	0	N	Δ	Y	Y
banana chips	1 oz	150	0	20	2	6	8	6	N	N	Δ	Y
berries: blackberries, gooseberries, loganberries, mulberries, raspberries	1 c	53-66	1-2	13-15	1-8	5-11	1	0	N	Y	Y	Y
blueberries	1/2c	41	1	11	2	7	0	0	N	Y	Y	Y
breadfruit	1/4 c	57	1	15	3	6	0	0	N	Δ	Y	Y
cantaloupe, honeydew	1 c	54-64	1	13-16	1	14	0	0	N	Δ	Y	Y
cherries, Barbados	1 c	31	0	8	1	n/a	0	0	N	Y	Y	Y
cherries, black, canned	1/4 c	44	1	11	1	10	0	0	N	Y	Y	Y
cherries, ground or red sour	1/2 c	37 - 44	1	8 - 11	1 -2	10	0	0	N	Y	Y	Y
cherries, Maraschino	7	70	0	21	0	21	0	0	N	N	Δ	Y
cherries, red, sour freeze-dried	.5 oz	60	1	12	0	n/a	0	0	N	Y	Y	Y
Clementine	1	40	1	9	2	6	0	0	N	Y	Y	Y
coconut, dried	2 tsp	55	0	2	0	1	5	5	N	Y	Y	Y
cranberries	1 c	44	0	12	4	4	0	0	N	Y	Y	Y
cranberries, dried	2 tbsp	45	0	11	1	10	0	0	N	Y	Y	Y
cranberry sauce, canned	1/2 slice	86	0	22	1	22	0	0	N	N	Δ	Y
currants, black, red, white	1/2c	31 - 35	1	8-9	2-4	4	0	0	N	Y	Y	Y
date, Chinese or deglet noor	1	22-23	0	6	1	5	0	0	N	Y	Y	Y
elderberries	1/4 c	26	0	7	3	n/a	0	0	N	Y	Y	Y
fig	1 medium	37	0	10	1	8	0	0	N	Y	Y	Y
Grapefruit: pink, red, white, other	1/2 medium	41-60	1	10-16	1-6	9-10	0	0	Y	Y	Y	Y
grapes: black, champagne, concord, green, red, seedless	1/2 c	50-61	1	13-16	1	12-15	0	0	N	Δ	Y	Y
kiwifruit	1 medium	46	1	11	2	7	0	0	N	Y	Y	Y
kumquat	3 oz	60	2	14	6	7	1	0	N	Y	Y	Y
lemon	1	15	0	5	1	1	0	0	Y	Y	Y	Y
lime	1	20	0	7	2	1	0	0	N	Y	Y	Y
mango	1/2	67	1	18	2	15	0	0	N	Δ	Y	Y
melons: cantaloupe, honeydew, muskmelon	1 c / 1/4 melon	54-64	1	13-16	1	14	0	0	N	Δ	Y	Y
nectarine	1 medium	70	1	17	1	13	0	0	N	Y	Y	Y
orange	1 medium	70	1	16	3	12	0	0	Y	Y	Y	Y
papaya	1 small	59	1	15	3	9	0	0	N	Y	Y	Y
peach	1 medium	38	1	9	1	8	0	0	N	Y	Y	Y
pear, persimmon	1/2 medium	50-59	0-1	13-16	2-4	9-11	0-1	0	N	Y	Y	Y
pineapple	1/2 c	37	0	10	1	7	0	0	N	Y	Y	Y
plantain chips	.5 oz	74	0	8	1	n/a	5	4	N	Y	Y	Y

Food/Item	Serving Size	Calories	Pro	Carb	Fiber	Sugar	Fat	Sat Fat	500 Diet	1st 3 wks	2nd 3 wks	Life
Fruit (cont)												
plum	1 medium	30	0	8	1	7	0	0	N	Y	Y	Y
pomegranate	1/2 of 3 3/8"	53	0	13	0	13	0	0	N	Δ	Y	Y
prunes	3 medium	50	1	13	2	6	0	0	N	Y	Y	Y
raisins: golden, purple	2 Tbsp	49-65	1	12-16	1	10-15	0	0	N	Δ	Y	Y
rhubarb	1 c	26	1	6	2	1	0	0	N	Y	Y	Y
star fruit	1 c	33	1	7	3	4	0	0	N	Y	Y	Y
strawberries	1/2 c	23	.5	5.5	1.5	3.5	0	0	Y	Y	Y	Y
tangelo, tangerine (mandarin orange)	1 medium	45-50	1	11-13	2-3	8	0-1	0-1	Y	Y	Y	Y
watermelon	1 c	45	1	11	1	9	0	0	N	Δ	Y	Y

Vegetables

Food/Item	Serving Size	Calories	Pro	Carbs	Fiber	Sugar	Fat	Sat Fat	500 Diet	1st 3 wks	2nd 3 wks	Life
alfalfa sprouts	1/2 c	5	1	1	1	0	0	0	N	Y	Y	Y
artichoke	1 medium	60	4	13	7	3	0	0	N	Δ	Y	Y
artichoke hearts (marinated or not), cooked	1/2 c	58	2	7	2	0	3	0	N	Y	Y	Y
arugula	4 oz	28	3	4	2	2	1	0	N	Δ	Y	Y
asparagus, cooked	4 oz	25	3	5	2	1	0	0	Y	Y	Y	Y
bamboo shoots, cooked	5 oz	17	2	3	1	0	0	0	Y	Y	Y	Y
bamboo shoots, raw	1 c	41	4	8	3	5	0	0	N	Δ	Δ	Y
beet greens, raw	1 c	8	1	2	1	0	0	0	Y	Y	Y	Y
beets, cooked	1/2 c	37	1	8	2	7	0	0	N	N	Δ	Y
broccoflower	1 c	32	3	6	3	0	0	0	N	Y	Y	Y
broccoli	1 c	44	5	8	5	3	1	0	N	Y	Y	Y
Brussel Sprouts	1 c	38	3	8	3	2	0	0	N	Y	Y	Y
burdock root, cooked	1/2 c	55	1	13	1	2	0	0	N	Δ	Δ	Y
cabbage	1/8 head	27	1.5	6.5	2.5	3.5	0	0	Y	Y	Y	Y
carrots, raw or cooked	1/2 c	27	1	6	2	3	1	0	N	Y	Y	Y
cauliflower	1 c	34	3	7	5	2	0	0	N	Y	Y	Y
celery	1 c	17	1	4	2	1	0	0	Y	Y	Y	Y
cherry tomatoes	1 c	27	1	6	2	4	0	0	Y	Y	Y	Y
chicory root	1 c	66	1	16	2	N/A	0	0	N	N	Δ	Y
collard greens, cooked	1 c	49	4	9	5	1	1	0	N	Y	Y	Y
corn	1/2 c	66	2	15	2	2	1	0	N	N	Δ	Y
cowpeas, cooked	1/2 c	100	7	17	3	1	1	0	N	N	Δ	Y
cucumber	1 c	16	1	3	1	2	0	0	Y	Y	Y	Y
eggplant	1 c	35	1	9	2	3	0	0	N	Y	Y	Y
endive	1/2 head	44	3	9	8	1	1	0	N	Y	Y	Y
green beans	1 c	38	2	8	3	2	0	0	N	Y	Y	Y
kale, cooked	1 c	36	2	7	3	2	1	0	N	Y	Y	Y
lettuce: Bibb, Boston, butter head, iceberg, loose-leaf, romaine	5" or 1 c	21	2	4	2	2	0	0	Y	Y	Y	Y
mountain yam, cooked	1/2 c	59	1	14	1	N/A	0	0	N	N	Δ	Y

Food/Item	Serving Size	Calories	Pro	Carb	Fiber	Sugar	Fat	Sat Fat	500 Diet	1st 3 wks	2nd 3 wks	Life
Vegetables (cont)												
mung bean sprouts	1/2 c	16	2	3	1	2	0	0	N	Y	Y	Y
mushrooms: brown Italian, cremini, enoki, morel, pickled, porcini, portobello	4-5	15	2	3	0	1	0	0	N	Y	Y	Y
mushrooms: shitake	1/2 c	41	1	10	2	3	0	0	N	Δ	Δ	Y
mustard greens	1 c	15	2	3	2	1	0	0	N	Y	Y	Y
okra, cooked	1 c	52	4	11	5	5	1	0	N	Δ	Y	Y
onion: red, white, yellow	1 small	29	1	7	1	3	0	0	Y	Y	Y	Y
onion: pearl, cooked	1/2 c	60	1	14	1	4	0	0	N	N	Δ	Y
palm hearts, canned	1/2 c	20	2	3	2	N/A	0	0	N	Δ	Y	Y
parsnips, cooked	1/2 c	63	1	15	3	4	0	0	N	N	Δ	Y
peas: green	1/2 c	59	4	10	4	4	0	0	N	Δ	Y	Y
peas: snow, raw	1/2 c	13	1	2	1	1	0	0	N	Y	Y	Y
peas: snow, steamed or cooked	1/2 c	35	2	6	2	3	0	0	N	Y	Y	Y
peppers: banana, hot chili, hot green	1	12-18	1	2-4	1-2	1-2	0	0	N	Y	Y	Y
peppers: bell (green, red, yellow)	1 medium	30	1	7	2	4-5	0	0	N	Y	Y	Y
potatoes												
baked	1 small	115	2	27	5	1	0	0	N	N	Δ	Y
new	3 oz	54	2	11	3	1	0	0	N	N	Δ	Y
French fried	1 c	185	3	28	3	n/a	7	3	N	N	Δ	Δ
hash browns	1/2 c	103	1	14	1	1	5	1	N	N	Δ	Δ
mashed, with milk and butter or scalloped	1/2 c	105 - 119	2-4	13-18	2	2	4-5	2-3	N	N	Δ	Y
twice baked	5 oz	204	4	27	4	1	9	3	N	N	Δ	Y
pumpkin, canned	1/2 c	42	1	10	4	4	0	0	N	Δ	Y	Y
radish	1/2 c	7-15	0-1	0-1	0-1	0-1	0	0	Y	Y	Y	Y
rutabaga	1 small	69	2	16	5	11	0	0	N	N	Δ	Y
sauerkraut, canned	1 c	30	0	6	2	4	0	0	N	Y	Y	Y
seaweed kelp	1/2 c	18	0	4	0	0	0	0	N	Y	Y	Y
snap beans: green, yellow	1 c	27	1	7	4	3	0	0	N	Y	Y	Y
spinach, raw	1 c	11	1	2	1	N/A	0	0	Y	Y	Y	Y
spinach, cooked	1 c	41	5	7	4	1	0	0	Y	Y	Y	Y
squash: acorn, butternut, cooked	1/2 c	41	1	11	3	N/A	0	0	N	Δ	Δ	Y
squash: scallop, straight neck	1 c	25-38	1-2	5-8	2-4	1-2	0	0	N	Y	Y	Y
squash: summer	1 medium	31	2	7	2	4	0	0	N	Y	Y	Y
squash: spaghetti, crookneck, winter	1 c	36-42	1-2	7-10	2-3	2-4	0-1	0	N	Δ	Y	Y
sweet potato, baked, mashed or canned	1 small	95-106	1-2	22-25	3	6-9	0	0	N	N	Δ	Y
Swiss chard, cooked	1 c	35	3	7	4	2	0	0	N	Y	Y	Y
tomato: red, green, orange	1 medium	18-35	1	4-7	1	4-5	0-1	0	Y	Y	Y	Y
tomato paste	1 Tbsp	13	1	3	1	2	0	0	N	Y	Y	Y
tomato puree	1/2 c	43	2	10	2	5	0	0	N	N	Y	Y
turnip cubed	1 c	36	8	2	5	0	0	0	N	Y	Y	Y
yam, cooked	1/2 c	39	1	9	1	0	0	0	N	N	Δ	Y
zucchini	1 medium	35	2	7	2	3	0	0	N	Y	Y	Y

Beans and Legumes
('Starchy' vegetables w/protein, fiber, and fat – a combination food)

Food/Item	Serving Size	Calories	Pro	Carb	Fiber	Sugar	Fat	Sat Fat	500 Diet	1st 3 wks	2nd 3 wks	Life
adzuki beans, cooked	1/2 c	147	9	28	8	0	0	0	N	Δ	Y	Y
baked beans	1/3 c	113	4	21	4	4	0	0	N	Δ *	Δ	Y
bean sprouts, (mung beans)	1/2 c	13	1	3	1	2	0	0	N	Δ	Y	Y
black beans, cooked	1/2 c	114	8	20	7	0	1	0	N	Δ	Y	Y
black-eyed peas, cooked	1/2 c	92	6.5	16	3.5	2.5	.5	0	N	Δ *	Δ	Y
butter beans (lima), cooked	1/2 c	105	6	20	5	1	0	0	N	Δ	Y	Y
chickpeas (garbanzos)	1/2 c	134	7	22	6	4	2	0	N	Δ *	Δ	Y
chili beans	1/2 c	100	6	22	7	1	.5	0	N	Δ	Y	Y
French beans	1/2 c	114	6	21	8	0	1	0	N	Δ	Y	Y
edamame	1/2 c	90	8.5	8	4	1.5	4	.5	N	Y	Y	Y
hummus	1/8 c	56	3	6	1	0	3	0	N	Δ	Δ	Y
kidney beans	1/2 c	110	8	20	8	0	0	0	N	Δ	Y	Y
lentils	1/4 c	161	13	28	11	3	1	0	N	Δ *	Δ	Y
mung beans, cooked	1/2 c	106	7	19	8	2	0	0	N	Δ	Y	Y
navy beans, cooked	1/2 c	127	7	24	20	0	1	0	N	Δ	Y	Y
pinto beans, cooked	1/2 c	122	8	22	8	0	1	0	N	Δ	Y	Y
refried beans	1/2 c	119	7	20	7	0	2	1	N	Δ	Y	Y
soybean sprouts, raw	1/2 c	24	3	2	0	0	1	0	N	Δ	Y	Y
soybean sprouts, steamed	1/2 c	38	4	3	0	0	2	0	N	Δ	Y	Y
soybeans, cooked	1/2 c	148	14	8	5	3	7	1	N	Δ *	Δ	Y
soybeans, dry roasted	1/4 c	202	15	14	8	0	11	2	N	Δ	Y	Y
split peas, cooked	1/2 c	116	8	21	8	3	0	0	N	Δ *	Δ	Y

Nuts, Nut Butters, and Seeds (Generally Fat & Protein – a combination food)

Food/Item	Serving Size	Calories	Pro	Carb	Fiber	Sugar	Fat	Sat Fat	500 Diet	1st 3 wks	2nd 3 wks	Life
almond butter: chocolate or plain	1 tbsp	90-101	2-3	3-5	1-2	1-2	8-9	1	N	Δ	Y	Y
almond paste	1 tbsp	65	1	7	1	5	4	0	N	Δ	Y	Y
almonds: dry-roasted, natural	1 oz	169	6	5.5	3.4	1.1	15	1.2	N	Δ	Y	Y
brazil nut butter	1 tbsp	95	2	2	1	n/a	10	2	N	Δ	Y	Y
brazil nuts, dried	1 oz	186	4	3.6	1.5	0	19	4.9	N	Δ	Y	Y
cashew butter: orange, or plain	1 tbsp	83-94	3	4-6	0-1	1	6-8	1-2	N	Δ	Y	Y
cashews, dry roasted	1 oz	163	4.3	9	1	0	13	3	N	N	Δ	Y
chestnuts: Chinese, European	1 oz	67-69	1	15	0-1.5	0-1	0-1	0	N	Δ	Y	Y
coconut: dried or fresh (unsweet)	1 tbsp	18	0	1	0	0	3	1	N	Y	Y	Y
flax seeds	1 tbsp	45	1	1	1	0	4	0	N	Y	Y	Y
hazelnut butter	1 tbsp	90	3	3	2	n/a	8	1	N	Δ	Y	Y
hazelnuts (filberts)	1 oz	178	4	5	3	0	17	1	N	Δ	Y	Y
macadamia nuts, dry-roasted	1 oz	203	2	3.6	2.3	1	22	3.4	N	Δ	Y	Y
mixed nuts, dry-roasted	1 oz	168	5	7	2.5	0	15	2	N	Δ	Y	Y
peanut butter, creamy or crunchy	1 tbsp	94	4	3	1	1	8	2	N	Δ	Y	Y
peanuts, dry-roasted, salted	1 oz	166	7	6	2	0	14	2	N	Δ	Y	Y
pecans or walnuts	1 oz	185-196	3-4	4	2-3	1	19-20	2	N	Δ	Y	Y

Dairy Products

(mostly protein and fat 'combination food')
i.e. Cheese, Cream, Yogurt

Food/Item	Serving Size	Calories	Pro	Carb	Fiber	Sugar	Fat	Sat Fat	500 Diet	1st 3 wks	2nd 3 wks	Life
cheese												
American, pasteurized	1" cube	24-68	4	0-2	0	0-2	0-6	0-4	N	Δ	Y	Y
blue, crumbled	1 Tbsp	30	2	0	0	0	2	2	N	Δ	Y	Y
Brie, Camembert, Cheddar, Colby, feta, fontina, Gruyere, Jalapeno Jack, Mexican queso asadero, Mexican queso chihuahua, Monterey Jack, mozzarella, Muenster, Parmesan, pepper Jack, provolone, Swiss	1" cube	45-69	3-8	0-2	0-1	0-1	2-6	0-4	N	Δ	Y	Y
cottage cheese, large/small curd	1/4 c	58	7	2	0	0	3	2	Y	Y	Y	Y
cottage cheese, low-fat 2%	1/4 c	50	7	3	0	3	1	1	N	Δ	Y	Y
cream cheese	2 Tbsp	101	2	1	0	0	10	6	N	Δ	Y	Y
cream cheese fat free	2 Tbsp	28	4	2	0	0	0	0	N	Δ	Y	Y
goat, Gouda, Roquefort	1 oz	76-128	5-9	0-10		0-1	6-10	4-7	N	Δ	Y	Y
Parmesan, grated	2 Tbsp	40	4	0	0	0	3	2	N	Δ	Y	Y
ricotta	1/4 c	108	7	2	0	0	8	5	N	Δ	Y	Y
Romano	2 Tbsp	70	6	0	0	0	5	3	N	Δ	Y	Y
string	1 oz	50	8	1	8	8	2	1	N	Δ	Y	Y
cream, light or heavy	1 Tbsp	29-51	0	0-1	0	0	3-6	2-3	N	Δ	Y	Y
cream, sour	1 Tbsp	31	0	1	0	0	3	2	N	Δ	Y	Y
half-and-half/cream substitute	1 Tbsp	20-32	0	1-3	0	0-3	1-2	1-2	N	Δ	Y	Y
topping, ex. Cool Whip	2 Tbsp	10-25	0	1-4	0	1-2	0-2	0-2	N	Δ	Y	Y
yogurt, plain, low-fat or fat free	4 oz	69-80	4-7	5-10	0	5-9	0-4	0-2	N	Δ	Y	Y
yogurt, flavored, low-fat	4 oz	90-141	3-6	16-24	0	16-21	1-3	0-2	N	N	Δ	Y
yogurt, flavored, fat free	4 oz	49-127	3-6	9-27	0-1	7-22	0	0	N	N	Δ	Y
yogurt, drink	4 oz	102	5	18	0	17	2	1	N	N	Δ	Y

Starches

bread, crackers, cereal, desserts, flour, grains, rice, sweet treats, snacks

Food/Item	Serving Size	Calories	Pro	Carbs	Fiber	Sugar	Fat	Sat Fat	500 Diet	1st 3 wks	2nd 3 wks	Life
Breads and Crackers												
bagel	1 oz	73 - 81	3	15-16	1-3	1	0-1	0	N	N	Δ	Δ
biscuit	1/2 of 2.5 inch	58-105	1-2	9-13	1-9	0-1	1-5	0-1	N	N	Δ	Δ
bread, regular	1 slice	65-90	1-4	12-20	1-3	0-2	0-2	0	N	N	Δ	Δ
bread crumbs	1 oz	109-112	2-4	14-20	1	1-2	1-2	0	N	N	Δ	Δ
bread stuffing	2 oz	100	2	12	2	2	4	0	N	N	Δ	Δ
corn bread	1 oz	89	2	14	1	N/A	3	1	N	N	Δ	Δ
corn bread stuffing	2 oz	102	2	12	2	2	4	2	N	N	Δ	Δ
cracker	.75 oz	73-93	1-3	15-18	1-4	0-5	0-4	0-1	N	N	Δ	Δ
cracker, graham	1 square	30	0	5	0	2	1	0	N	N	Δ	Y
crispbread, Wasa	1 slice	30-60	1-2	9-14	0-3	0-1	0-2	0	N	N	Δ	Δ
croissant	1 medium	232	4	26	2	6	12	6	N	N	Δ	Δ
English muffin	1/2 muffin	65-78	2-3	13-15	1-2	0-4	0-1	0	N	N	Δ	Δ
French toast	1/2 slice	74	3	8	0	N/A	4	1	N	N	Δ	Δ
hush puppy	1 oz	93	2	13	1	N/A	4	1	N	N	Δ	Δ
muffin	1 oz	53-107	1-2	10-16	1	3-13	0-5	0-1	N	N	Δ	Δ
pancake	1 oz	43-85	1-2	7-14	0-1	0-4	0-2	0	N	N	Δ	Δ
roll, cinnamon	1 oz	112	2	15	1	10	5	1	N	N	Δ	Δ
roll, dinner	1 oz	75-84	2-3	11-15	0-2	0-2	1-2	0-1	N	N	Δ	Δ
roll, hamburger/hot dog bun	1/2 bun	60	3	11	1	2	1	1	N	N	Δ	Δ
taco shell	5 in. shell	50-62	1	7-8	0-1	0	2-3	0-1	N	N	Δ	Δ
tortilla, corn	6 in.	57	1	12	2	0	1	0	N	N	Δ	Δ
tortilla, flour	6 in.	100	3	16	1	1	2	1	N	N	Δ	Δ
waffle	1 (1 oz)	70-95	2-8	8-15	1-4	1-4	1-6	0-1	N	N	Δ	Δ

Cereal

Cereals, in general, are clear starches without much benefit (fiber or protein), but there are good exceptions to the rule. A few of the good exceptions are listed below, but the list is always changing, so look for high protein and high fiber for the best options.

Food/Item	Serving Size	Calories	Pro	Carbs	Fiber	Sugar	Fat	Sat Fat	500 Diet	1st 3 wks	2nd 3 wks	Life
cereal (non puffed), cold or hot	1/4-1 c	74-210	1-8	9-47	1-14	0-20	0-7	0-1	N	N	Δ	Y
cereal (puffed)	1 c	42-60	1-8	0-6	0-1	0	0	0-1	N	N	Δ	Y
cereal, healthier choices (high protein & fiber)												
All-bran	1 c	153	9	45	18	9	3	0	N	N	Δ	Y
Bob's Red Mill, hot cereals	1/4 - 1/3 c	110-180	4-8	20-35	3-10	0-1	1-5	0-1	N	N	Δ	Y
Ezekial 4:9 : almond, golden flax, original	1/2 c	180-200	7-8	37-41	5-6	<1	1-2.5	0	N	N	Δ	Y
Kashi: GoLean, Good Friends, Heart to Heart	1/2 - 3/4 c	85-110	3-5	18-25	4-6	5-6	1-2	0	N	N	Δ	Y
oat bran	1/2 c	116	8	32	8	0	4	0	N	N	Δ	Y
oatmeal, old-fashioned, dry	1/4 c	74	3	14	2	0	2	0	N	N	Δ	Y

67

Food/Item	Serving Size	Calories	Pro	Carbs	Fiber	Sugar	Fat	Sat Fat	500 Diet	1st 3 wks	2nd 3 wks	Life
Cereal (cont.)												
puffed millet	1 c	60	2	11	1	0	0	1	N	N	Y	Y
shredded wheat cereal	1 serving	85	3	21	3	0	0	0	N	N	Y	Y
Special K	1 c	118	6	22	0	4	0	0	N	N	Δ	Y
Special K Low Carb Lifestyle Protein Plus	1 c	134	14	18	6	2	4	0	N	N	Y	Y

Grains and Rice

Food/Item	Serving Size	Calories	Pro	Carbs	Fiber	Sugar	Fat	Sat Fat	500 Diet	1st 3 wks	2nd 3 wks	Life
amaranth, barley, buckwheat, buckwheat flour, bulgar, couscous, corn flour, corn grits, cornmeal, cornstarch, hominy, quinoa, rice bran, rice flour, rye flour, semolina, sorghum flour, tapioca, triticale flour, wheat flour	serving size varies, see package	42-91	1-4	10-17	1-4	0-1	0-2	0	N	N	Δ	Y
almond flour/meal	1/4 c	145	5	4	3	1	12	1	N	Δ	Δ	Y
coconut flour	2 Tbsp	26	2	10	9	0	1.5	1	N	Δ	Y	Y
millet, cooked	1/4 c	52	2	10	1	0	0	0	N	N	Δ	Y
oat bran, cooked	1/3 c	29	2	8	2	n/a	1	0	N	N	Δ	Y
pasta, (basically all varieties)	1 c	140-600	6-14	30-75	1-6	0-6	2-20	0-16	N	N	Δ	Δ
rice: white or brown; short, medium, long grain; wild or not; cooked	1/4 c	42 - 60	1	9-13	0-1	0-1	0	0	N	N	Δ	Y
vital wheat gluten	.5 oz	52	11	2	0	0	0	0	N	Y	Y	Y
wheat germ	2 Tbsp	52	3	7	2	n/a	1	0	N	N	Δ	Y

Desserts and Sweet Treats: candy, cookies, cake (Generally Starch and Sugar)

Food/Item	Serving Size	Calories	Pro	Carbs	Fiber	Sugar	Fat	Sat Fat	500 Diet	1st 3 wks	2nd 3 wks	Life
brownie	2" square	112	1	12	1	8	7	2	N	N	Δ	Δ
brownie, fat-free or low-fat	2" square	100-107	2-5	19-20	1	14-16	0-1	0-1	N	N	Δ	Δ
cake												
angel food	1 serving	120	3	27	0	20	0	0	N	N	Δ	Y
cake with icing: white, chocolate, yellow	1 serving	275-425	2-5	35-61	0-1	25-45	10-16	3-6	N	N	Δ	Δ
cake without icing: white, chocolate, yellow	1 serving	187-225	2-5	36-42	0-1	26-29	9-11	1-2	N	N	Δ	Δ
cake, pound, fat free	1 oz	80	2	17	0	10	0	0	N	N	Δ	Y
cake, pound, regular	1 serving	290	5	39	1	21	13	7	N	N	Δ	Δ
cheesecake	1 serving	309	8	30	0	21	18	9	N	N	Δ	Δ
cheesecake, fat-free	1 serving	140	7	28	1	18	0	0	N	N	Δ	Y
candy												
bars: 3 Musketeers, 5th Avenue, Almond Joy, Baby Ruth, M & Ms, Milky Way, Mounds, Nestle Crunch, Snickers, Twix	fun size	50 - 108	1-2	5-14	0-1	4 - 13	2 - 6	1-2	N	N	Δ	Δ
chocolate covered almonds	5	90	1	10	1	5	5	5	N	N	Δ	Y
chocolate covered peanuts	5	105	5	10	1	10	5	5	N	N	Δ	Y
chocolate covered raisin	5	25	0	5	1	5	0	0	N	N	Δ	Y
gum, regular	1 stick	10	0	3	0	1	0	0	N	N	Δ	Y
gum, sugar-free	1 stick	2	0	1	0	0	0	0	N	Y	Y	Y
hard, sugar-free	1 piece	11	0	3	0	0	0	0	N	Δ	Y	Y
Hershey's Kisses	3 piece	78	0	9	0	6	3	3	N	N	Δ	Y

Food/Item	Serving Size	Calories	Pro	Carbs	Fiber	Sugar	Fat	Sat Fat	500 Diet	1st 3 wks	2nd 3 wks	Life
Dessert and Sweet Treats (cont): candy												
licorice, black or red vine	1 piece	35	0	8-9	0	4-5	0	0	N	N	Δ	Y
Peppermint Patty	fun size	10	0	2	0	2	0	0	N	N	Δ	Y
Reese's Peanut Butter Cup	fun size	36	1	4	0	3	2	1	N	N	Δ	Y
Rolo	3 pieces	42	0	6	0	6	3	0	N	N	Δ	Δ
Skittles, Starburst	1 oz	112-115	0	24-26	0	19-22	1-2	0	N	N	Δ	Δ
Tootsie Pop	1	60	0	15	0	10	0	0	N	N	Δ	Y
cookie												
animal cracker	5	40	0	5	0	1	0	0	N	N	Δ	Y
biscotti, chocolate-covered, sugar-free	1	40	1	6	0	0	2	1		N	N	Δ	Y
butter cookie	.5 oz	75	1	10	0	n/a	4	1	N	N	Δ	Δ
chocolate cookie	2.5 oz	210	2	30	1	20	10	4	N	N	Δ	Δ
chocolate chip, regular or sugar free	.5	62-78	1	9	0	0--7	4-5	1-2	N	N	Δ	Δ
chocolate sandwich, regular or reduced-fat	1	43-47	0-1	7-8	0	4	1-2	0	N	N	Δ	Δ
coconut macaroon	1	97	1	17	0	17	3	3	N	N	Δ	Δ
devil's food	1	72	1	15	n/a	n/a	1	1	N	N	Δ	Δ
devil's food, SnackWells fat-free	1	49	1	12	0	7	0	0	N	N	Δ	Y
fig bar, regular or whole grain	1	56-60	1	11-13	1	7-8	0-1	0	N	N	Δ	Y
fortune cookie	1	30	0	7	0	4	0	0	N	N	Δ	Y
gingersnap	1	29	0	5	0	1	1	0	N	N	Δ	Y
graham cracker	1 square	30	0	5	0	2	1	0	N	N	Δ	Y
lemon sandwich	1	156	1	8	1	3	2	0	N	N	Δ	Δ
oatmeal	1	106	2	17	1	8	4	1	N	N	Δ	Δ
oatmeal with raisin	1	107	1	17	1	9	4	1	N	N	Δ	Δ
oatmeal, sugar-free	1	50	1	7	1	0	2	1	N	N	Δ	Y
peanut butter	1	95	2	12	0	n/a	5	1	N	N	Δ	Y
peanut butter sandwich	1	67	1	9	0	5	3	1	N	N	Δ	Y
sugar, regular or fat free	1	71-98	1	17	0	8	0-3	0-1	N	N	Δ	Δ
sugar wafer	1	34	0	4	0	3	2	0	N	N	Δ	Y
vanilla wafer	1	18	0	3	n/a	1	1	0	N	N	Δ	Y
custard, 2% or whole milk	1/2 c	148-161	5	23	0	n/a	4-5	2-3	N	N	Δ	Y
donuts												
crème puff, chocolate w/custard	1 3"	293	7	27	1	7	18	5	N	N	Δ	Δ
cake, chocolate or plain	1	180-204	2-3	19-21	1	7-10	11-13	2-3	N	N	Δ	Δ
cake, sugared	1	310	4	28	1	10	20	4	N	N	Δ	Δ
donut, raised, glazed	1	160	3	23	1	5	7	2	N	N	Δ	Δ
donut, raised with crème filling	1	320	4	39	1	19	16	4	N	N	Δ	Δ
éclair with custard and chocolate	1	204	5	19	0	5	12	3	N	N	Δ	Δ
flan	1/2 c	150	4	25	0	n/a	4	2	N	N	Δ	Y
frozen yogurt												
chocolate, reg or fat-free	1/2 c	104-110	3-5	19-21	1-2	16-18	0-3	0-2	N	N	Δ	Y
coffee, strawberry fat-free, vanilla	1/2 c	140	5	20-31	0	18-27	0-5	0-3	N	N	Δ	Y
vanilla, fat-free	1/2 c	95	5	19	0	19	0	0	N	Δ	Y	Y

Food/Item	Serving Size	Calories	Pro	Carb	Fiber	Sugar	Fat	Sat Fat	500 Diet	1st 3 wks	2nd 3 wks	Life
Dessert and Sweet Treats: gelatin (cont)												
gelatin, fruit-flavored, regular	1/2 c	80	2	19	0	19	0	0	N	N	Δ	Y
gelatin, flavored, sugar free	1/2 c	20	2	0	0	0	0	0	N	Y	Y	Y
ice cream												
chocolate, low-fat	1/2 c	120	3	21	2	18	2	1	N	N	Δ	Y
chocolate, butter pecan	1/2 c	170-188	2-3	12-15	0-1	13	12-13	5-8	N	N	Δ	Y
strawberry	1/2 c	250	4	23	1	21	16	10	N	N	Δ	Δ
vanilla	1/2 c	133	2	16	0	14	7	4	N	N	Δ	Y
vanilla, low-fat	1/2 c	110	3	19	1	18	2	1	N	N	Δ	Y
vanilla, sugar-free	1/2 c	99	3	15	0	4	4	3	N	N	Y	Y
ice cream cone, sugar	1	60	1	12	0	4	.5	0	N	N	Y	Y
ice cream cone, wafer type	1	17	0	3	0	.2	0	0	N	Δ	Y	Y
ice cream novelties												
Creamsicle: all flavors, sugar-free	2 pops	40	1	10	6	0	2	1.5	N	Δ	Y	Y
Dreamsicle	1	91	2	18	n/a	n/a	2	1	N	Δ	Y	Y
Drumstick	1	159	3	18	n/a	n/a	9	4	N	Δ	Y	Y
Fudgsicle, fat-free	1	70	3	14	1	10	0	0	N	Δ	Y	Y
Fudgsicle, sugar-free	2 pops	70	4	16	4	0	2	1	N	Δ	Y	Y
Popsicle: all flavors, sugar-free	1	15	0	4	0	0	0	0	N	Y	Y	Y
sandwich	1	144	3	22	1	15	6	3	N	N	Δ	Y
sandwich, low fat	1	130	3	27	1	14	1	1	N	N	Δ	Y
Skinny Cow, fudge bar, fat-free	1	100	4	21	0	18	0	0	N	N	Δ	Y
Skinny Cow, sandwich, fat-free	1	140	4	30	5	4	2	1	N	N	Δ	Y
marshmallows, 1 large or 10 mini	2 or 20 mini	46	0	12	0	8	0	0	N	N	Δ	Y
pastry, Danish: cheese, cinnamon	1	266-280	5-6	26-30	1	5-17	16	4-5	N	N	Δ	Y
pastry, Danish: fruit	1	335	5	45	n/a	n/a	16	3	N	N	Δ	Y
pie												
banana cream	1 piece	387	6	47	1	23	20	5	N	N	Δ	Y
chocolate crème	1 piece	280	4	36	1	21	14	4	N	N	Δ	Y
coconut cream	1 piece	259	3	27	0	n/a	17	8	N	N	Δ	Y
egg custard	1 piece	221	6	22	2	12	12	2	N	N	Δ	Y
fruit: apple, blueberry, cherry, peach	1 piece	261 - 304	2	40-47	1-2	15-18	12-13	3-5	N	N	Δ	Y
fruit: lemon (no meringue)	1 piece	189	4	34	0	31	5	2	N	N	Δ	Y
lemon meringue	1 piece	303	2	53	1	37	10	2	N	N	Δ	Y
mince	1 piece	477	4	79	4	47	18	4	N	N	Δ	Y
mud	1 piece	244	3	37	2	28	10	7	N	N	Δ	Y
pecan	1 piece	503	6	64	n/a	n/a	27	5	N	N	Δ	Y
pumpkin, sweet potato	1 piece	295-316	6-7	36-41	2-4	n/a	14	3-5	N	N	Δ	Y
pumpkin, crustless, sugar-free	1 piece	62	4.6	7	3	4.3	1.8	0	N	Δ	Y	Y
pastry, Danish: fruit	1	335	5	45	n/a	n/a	16	3	N	N	Δ	Y
pudding, bread	1/2 c	237	7	33	1	20	8	4	N	N	Δ	Y
pudding, regular, cooked and instant packaged, all flavors	1/2 c	95-120	3	28	0	20	0	0	N	N	Δ	Y

Food/Item	Serving Size	Calories	Pro	Carbs	Fiber	Sugar	Fat	Sat Fat	500 Diet	1st 3 wks	2nd 3 wks	Life
Dessert and Sweet Treats: Pudding (cont)												
pudding, fat-free, cooked and instant packaged, all flavors	1/2 c	100	3	23	1	17	0	0	N	N	Δ	Y
pudding, fat-free, sugar-free, cooked and instant packaged, all flavors	1/2 c	25 - 35	0-1	6-8	0-1	0	0	0	N	Δ	Y	Y
pudding, plum	3 oz	235	4	42	2	30	6	n/a	N	N	Δ	Y
pudding, rice, fat-free	1/2 c	140	5	29	0	19	0	0	N	N	Δ	Y
pudding, sugar-free, cooked and instant packaged, all flavors	1/2 c	60-80	5	14	1	0	0	0	N	Δ	Δ	Y
pudding, whole milk	1/2 c	169	5	28	1	17	4	3	N	N	Δ	Y
sherbert: lemon mime orange	1/2 c	90-127	0-1	22-32	0-2	18-32	0-1	0-1	N	N	Δ	Y
sorbet, Ben & Jerry's: Berried Treasure, Strawberry Kiwi Swirl, Jamaican Me Crazy	1/2 c	110-130	0	28-33	1-4	24-28	0	0	N	N	Δ	Y
syrup: butterscotch, caramel, chocolate, fudge	1 tbsp	52 - 67	0-1	12-14	0-1	6-10	0-2	0-1	N	N	Δ	Y
syrup, sugar-free: caramel, chocolate	1 tbsp	0-10	0	0-4	0	0	0	0	N	Δ	Y	Y
tapioca, fat-free	1/2 c	111	2	26	0	20	0	0	N	N	Δ	Y
tapioca, whole milk	1/2 c	162	4	27	0	n/a	4	2	N	N	Δ	Y
topping: marshmallow, pineapple, strawberry	1 tbsp	54-60	0	14-15	0	4-6	0	0	N	N	Δ	Y

Snacks: chips, pretzels, popcorn (Generally a starch, but may be a sugar or both)												
baked: Cheetos, Doritos Nacho Cheese, Lays (Cheddar, BBQ, Original, Sour Cream and Onion), Ruffles Original, Tostitos	1 oz	110-130	2-3	19-24	0-2	0-3	1-5	0-1	N	N	Δ	Y
Cheese puff: crunchy and original bakes	1 oz	158-162	2	13-15	0-1	1	10-11	2-3	N	N	Δ	Y
Chex Party Mix	1 oz	123	3	21	1	2	3	1	N	N	Δ	Y
corn chips: regular, BBQ, French onion, whole grain	1 oz	140-150	2	16-19	0-2	0-3	6-9	1-6	N	N	Δ	Y
Corn nuts: BBQ, cheese, original, plain, ranch	1 oz	122-132	2-3	19-20	2	n/a-0	4-5	1	N	N	Δ	Y
Fruit Roll-ups: cherry, grape, strawberry	1 oz	52-53	0	12	0	5	1	0	N	N	Δ	Y
Gold Fish crackers	25 fish	65	1	10	1	3	3	1	N	N	Δ	Y
granola bar												
almond, banana nut, chocolate chip	1	95-117	2	14-15	1	6	4-6	1-3	N	N	Δ	Y
carob chip	1	80	2	15	1	7	2	0	N	N	Δ	Y
fat free: blueberry, chocolate chip, , raisin, raspberry, strawberry	1	140	2	35	3	14	0	0	N	N	Δ	Y
low-fat: almond, apple-cinnamon, chocolate chip, chocolate chunk, Dutch apple, honey nut, oatmeal, oatmeal raisin, peanut crunch, s'mores, wild berry	1	82-111	1-2	16-22	1	0-10	2-3	0-1	N	N	Δ	Y

Food/Item	Serving Size	Calories	Pro	Carbs	Fiber	Sugar	Fat	Sat Fat	500 Diet	1st 3 wks	2nd 3 wks	Life
Snacks: chips, pretzels, popcorn (continued)												
vanilla yogurt (granola bar)	1	140	2	26	1	13	4	2	N	N	Δ	Y
jerky (protein; not sugar or starch)												
Beef	1 oz	126	9	3	3	0	8	3	N	Δ	Y	Y
teriyaki, turkey	1 oz	81	13-14	3-5	0	1-3	1	0	N	Δ	Y	Y
Venison	1 oz	96	10	4	0	0	4	2	N	Y	Y	Y
Popcorn												
air-popped	1 c	31	1	6	1	0	0	0	N	N	Δ	Y
Caramel	1 oz	122	1	22	1	15	4	1	N	N	Δ	Y
caramel, fat-free	1 oz	108	1	26	1	18	0	0	N	N	Δ	Y
original, kettle	1 c	80	1	16	2	10	1	0	N	N	Δ	Y
oil-popped	1 c	55	1	6	1	0	3	1	N	N	Δ	Y
pork skins: plain or BBQ	0.5 oz	76-77	8-9	0	0	0	4-5	2	N	Y	Y	Y
potato chips												
baked: plain, BBQ	1 oz	112-120	2	18-22	2	2	4	0	N	N	Δ	Y
fat-free: plain	1 oz	108	2	24	2	2	0	0	N	N	Δ	Y
reduced-fat or light: Cheddar cheese, Jalapeno, BBQ, plain	1 oz	140-150	2	18	2	0-2	8	0-2	N	N	Δ	Y
regular: BBQ, plain, sour cream	1 oz	140	2	14	2	n/a	10	2	N	N	Δ	Y
Pretzel												
hard: rods, sticks, twists	1 oz	100	4	24	2	2	0	0	N	N	Δ	Y
soft: almond, cinnamon sugar, garlic, original, sesame, sour cream & onion	1 medium	310-350	9-11	63-74	2-4	9-16	1-8	0-5	N	N	Δ	Y
rice cake, most flavors	1	34-35	0-1	7	0	0	0	0	N	N	Δ	Y
rice cake: banana nut, chocolate crunch, cinnamon streusel, honey nut, lemon , multigrain, peanut butter, popcorn, seaweed	1	50-83	1-2	11-18	0-1	1-5	0-1	0	N	N	Δ	Y
sesame stick	1 oz	144	4	14	0	0	10	2	N	N	Δ	Y
taro chips (regular or sweet potato)	1 oz	140-142	0-2	18-20	2-4	2	8	2	N	N	Δ	Y
tortilla chips												
baked: light or low-fat	1 oz	110-126	2-4	20-24	2	0	2-4	0	N	N	Δ	Y
Regular	1 oz	142	2	18	2	0	7	1	N	N	Δ	Y
trail mix -- varies by brand/type												
trail mix, Kirkland	1/4 c	140	2	18	1	14	6	1	N	N	Δ	Y
trail mix, organic fruit and nuts, Trader Joe's	1 oz	130	8	12	3	n/a	8	2	N	Δ	Y	Y
trail mix, Nature (Wal-Mart brand)	1/4 c	149	8	10	5	5	9	1	N	N	Y	Y
wasabi peas, Trader Joe's	1/3 c	80	1	12	1	4	3	1	N	N	Δ	Y

Condiments
(Watch for Sugar/Carbs)

Food/Item	Serving Size	Calories	Pro	Carb	Fiber	Sugar	Fat	Sat Fat	500 Diet	1st 3 wks	2nd 3 wks	Life
barbeque sauce (check label)	1 packet	6-25	0	1-7.5	0	1-6	0	0	N	Δ	Y	Y
barbeque sauce, low sugar	1 tbsp	5	0	2	0	0	0	0	N	Y	Y	Y
capers, drained	1 tbsp	2	0	0	0	0	0	0	N	Y	Y	Y
fruit spreads: apricot, blackberry, black cherry, blueberry, boysenberry, concord grape, harvest berry, orange, peach, plum marmalade, raspberry, strawberry	1 tbsp	38-40	0-1	10	0-1	8-10	0	0	N	N	Δ	Y
Horseradish	1 tbsp	7	0	2	0	1	0	0	N	Y	Y	Y
horseradish: cream, mustard, sauce	1 tbsp	29-30	0-1	1-2	0-1	0-1	2-3	0-2	N	Δ	Y	Y
jam/jelly, all flavors, regular	1 tbsp	50-56	0	13-14	0-1	10-12	0	0	N	N	Δ	Y
jam/jelly, all flavors, low sugar	1 tbsp	25	0	5-6	0	5-6	0	0	N	N	Y	Y
jam/jelly, sugar free	1 tbsp	10	0	5	0	0	0	0	N	N	Y	Y
Ketchup	1 tbsp	15	0	4	0	3	0	0	N	Δ	Y	Y
Mayonnaise	1 tbsp	100	0	0	0	0	11	1-2	N	Y	Y	Y
mayonnaise, light	1 tbsp	46-50	0	1-2	0	0-1	5	1	N	Y	Y	Y
Mustard , plain (*check ingredients for 500 calorie phase)	1 tbsp	10	1	1	0	0	0	0	Y*	Y	Y	Y
mustard, honey	1 tbsp	21	1	4	1	3	0	0	N	Δ	Y	Y
olives, black	5 large	25	0	1	1	0	2	0	N	Y	Y	Y
olives, green	5	50	0	3	0	0	5	0	N	Y	Y	Y
pickle, bread butter	1/4 cup	34	0	8	1	4	0	0	N	N	Δ	Y
pickle, dill	1 med	12	0	3	1	2	0	0	N	Δ	Y	Y
pickle, sweet	1 med	29	0	8	0	4	0	0	N	N	Δ	Y
pickle relish	1 tbsp	14-19	0	4-5	0	3-5	0	0	N	Δ	Δ	Y
salad dressing - extreme variances												
salad dressing with 0 carbs, 0 sugar and 0 fat (i.e. homemade vinegar w/stevia or similar)	2 tbsp	0-10	0	0	0	0	0	0	Δ	Y	Y	Y
salad dressing with 3 or less carbs, less than 2 sugars and 12 or less fats: most ranch, blue cheese, vinaigrette, Italian	2 tbsp	0 - 120	0-1	0-3	0-1	0-2	0-12	0-2.5	N	Δ	Δ	Y
salad dressing with more than 3 carbs, more than 3 sugars and/or more than 12 fats: examples: French (Catalina Light Done Right of Original), honey mustard, honey Dijon, some balsamic vinaigrettes	2 tbsp	60 - 160	0-1	1- 15	0-1	1-9	1-17	0-2.5	N	N	Δ	Y
salsa: picante, red jalapeno, thick and chunky, regular	1 tbsp	4	0	1	0	1	0	0	N	Y	Y	Y
salsa, black bean and corn	2 tbsp	15	1	3	0	1	0	0	N	Y	Y	Y
soy sauce	1 tbsp	11	2	1	0	0	0	0	N	Y	Y	Y
steak sauce	1 tbsp	5	0	1	0	0	0	0	N	Y	Y	Y
tartar sauce	1 tbsp	70	0	1	0	0	8	1	N	N	Y	Y
tartar sauce, low calorie	1 tbsp	31	0	2	0	0	3	0	N	Δ	Y	Y
vinaigrette: balsamic, barbeque, Italian, red wine	1 tbsp	25-45	0	2	0	0-2	2-5	0-1	N	Δ	Y	Y
vinaigrette: basil, Greek, herb	1 tbsp	55-85	0	1-13	0	0-2	6-9	1	N	Δ	Y	Y

Condiments (cont)
(Watch for Sugar/Carbs)

Food/Item	Serving Size	Calories	Pro	Carb	Fiber	Sugar	Fat	Sat Fat	500 Diet	1st 3 wks	2nd 3 wks	Life
vinegar: apple cider, cider, distilled, garlic wine, Italian herb, malt, red wine organic, rice, tarragon, white distilled	1 tbsp	0-3	0	0-1	0	0	0	0	Y	Y	Y	Y
vinegar: balsamic, brown rice, champagne, golden balsamic, rice seasoned, white wine	1 tbsp	5-12	0	0-3	0	0-2	0	0	Δ	Y	Y	Y
Wasabi	1 tbsp	2	0	0	0	0	0	0	Y	Y	Y	Y
Worcestershire sauce	1 tbsp	11	0	3	0	0	2	0	N	Y	Y	Y
Worcestershire sauce, low sodium	1 tbsp	5	0	1	0	1	0	0	N	Y	Y	Y

Fats and Oils

Food/Item	Serving Size	Calories	Pro	Carb	Fiber	Sugar	Fat	Sat Fat	500 Diet	1st 3 wks	2nd 3 wks	Life
bacon grease	1 tsp	39	0	0	0	0	4	2	N	Δ	Y	Y
butter, regular or light	1 tsp	24-33	0	0	0	0	3-4	2	N	Δ	Y	Y
cooking spray	1 serving	0	0	0	0	0	0	0	N	Δ	Y	Y
oil: cod, cod liver, salmon, flaxseed, ghee, lard, margarine, almond, avocado, canola, canola and soybean, cocoa butter, coconut, corn and canola, cottonseed, grapeseed, hazelnut, mustard, olive, palm, peanut, safflower, sesame, soybean, walnut, wheat germ	1 tsp	34-41	0	0	0	0	4-5	0-4	N	Δ	Y	Y
oil, cashew nut	1 tbsp	47	1	2	0	0	4	1	N	Δ	Y	Y

Sweeteners

Food/Item	Serving Size	Calories	Pro	Carb	Fiber	Sugar	Fat	Sat Fat	500 Diet	1st 3 wks	2nd 3 wks	Life
agave nectar (lower glycemic index and takes less than sugar)	1 tsp	15	0	4	0	4	0	0	N	Δ	Δ	Y
aspartame: NutraSweet, Equal	1 serving	0	0	<1	0	0	0	0	N	Y	Y	Y
brown sugar, unpacked	1 tsp	11	0	3	0	3	0	0	N	N	Δ	Y
cane sugar, organic, unrefined	1 tsp	16	0	4	0	4	0	0	N	N	Δ	Y
corn syrup, light or dark	1 tsp	19-20	0	5	0	2	0	0	N	N	Δ	Y
fructose, dry	1 tsp	15	0	4	0	4	0	0	N	N	Δ	Y
honey	1 tsp	21	0	6	0	5	0	0	N	N	Δ	Y
Lakanto (all-natural), Fermented Erythritol, Luo Han Guo	1 tsp	0	0	4	0	0	0	0	N	Y	Y	Y
maple syrup, molasses, light/dark	1 tsp	17-20	0	4-5	0	4-5	0	0	N	N	Δ	Y
powdered sugar	1 tsp	10	0	2	0	2	0	0	N	N	Δ	Y
saccharin: Sweet'N Low, Sweet Twin, and Necta Sweet	1 serving	0	0	<1	0	0	0	0	Y	Y	Y	Y
sorghum syrup	1 tsp	17	0	4	0	4	0	0	N	N	Δ	Y
sucralose: Splenda	1 serving	0	0	<1	0	0	0	0	N	Y	Y	Y
stevia	1 packet	0	0	1	0	0	0	0	Y	Y	Y	Y
Sugar Twin	1 packet	0	0	<1	0	0	0	0	Y	Y	Y	Y
white sugar	1 tsp	16	0	4	0	4	0	0	N	N	Δ	Y

Herbs and Spices

Food/Item	Serving Size	Calories	Pro	Carb	Fiber	Sugar	Fat	Sat Fat	500 Diet	1st 3 wks	2nd 3 wks	Life
The following herbs and spices vary in serving size. All are allowed on all phases of the protocol as long as no sugars or oils (in ANY form) are listed in the ingredients -- you can NOT go by the nutritional information label as it may not reflect small amounts of sugar(s) and oil(s). Allspice, almond extract, anise seed, annatto, asafetida, basil, bay leaves, borage, caraway seed, cardamom seed, celery salt, celery seed, chervil, chicory, chili powder, chives, cilantro, cinnamon, cloves, cocoa powder (unsweetened), coriander, cumin seed, curry (fresh or powder), dill seed, dill weed, epazote, fennel seed, fenugreek (leaves or seed), five-spice powder (Chinese), galangal (Thai ginger), garlic powder, garlic salt, ginger, gingerroot, Italian seasoning, jerk seasoning, lemongrass, lemon pepper seasoning, mace, marjoram, Mexican seasoning blend, mustard seed, nutmeg, onion powder, oregano, paprika, parsley, pepper (black, ground, cayenne, chili flakes, white), peppermint, poppy seed, poultry seasoning, pumpkin pie spice, rosemary, saffron, sage, salt, salt substitute, savory, sesame seed, spearmint, tarragon, turmeric, vanilla extract.	1 serving; usually 1/4 tsp	0-5	0-1	<1	0	<1	<.5	0	Y	Y	Y	Y
Many commercial seasonings have sugar and/or oils. The nutritional label may not reflect these ingredients, so the actual ingredient list should be reviewed. Some popular examples are Grill Creations Italian Herb, Lowery's Seasoning Salt, McCormick California Garlic Salt and Hot Shot! Ortega Fiesta Mexican Seasoning	varies	0-20	0-2	0-5	0-1	0-4	0-2	0	N	Δ	Y	Y
Any seasoning with more than 4 grams of sugar per serving.	varies	10	>0	>0	>0	>4	>0	>0	N	N	Δ	Y

Sauces and Gravy

Food/Item	Serving Size	Calories	Pro	Carb	Fiber	Sugar	Fat	Sat Fat	500 Diet	1st 3 wks	2nd 3 wks	Life
gravy												
au jus	2 tbsp	5	0	1	0	n/a	n/a	0	N	Y	Y	Y
beef, chicken, mushroom, pork, sausage, turkey	1 tbsp	7-24	0-1	1	0	n/a - 0	n/a - 0	0-2	N	Δ	Y	Y
biscuit	1 tbsp	77	0	9	0	0	5	0	N	N	Δ	Y
sauces												
Alfredo	2 tbsp	55	1	1	0	0	5	2	N	Δ	Y	Y
BBQ	2 tbsp	24	0	4	0	2	0	0	N	Δ	Y	Y
basil pesto, Melissa's	2 tbsp	170	3	2	0	1	17	3	N	Δ	Y	Y
béarnaise	2 tbsp	78	0	0	0	0	8	4	N	Δ	Y	Y
cheese	2 tbsp	60	3	2	0	.5	5	2	N	Δ	Y	Y
chili	1 tbsp	20	0	5	0	4	0	0	N	N	Y	Y
Creole	1/4 c	25	1	4	1	3	1	0	N	Y	Y	Y
curry	1 tbsp	9	0	0	0	0	1	0	N	Y	Y	Y
enchilada	1/4 c	25	.5	3	0	1	1	0	N	Δ	Y	Y
hoi sin	1 tbsp	24	1	7	0	4	1	0	N	Δ	Y	Y
hollandaise	1 tbsp	43	1	0	0	0	5	3	N	Δ	Y	Y
marinara	1 tbsp	9	0	1	0	0	0	0	N	Y	Y	Y
marinara, spaghetti	1/4 c	57	1.5	8	2	0	2	0	N	Δ	Y	Y
mole verde	1 tbsp	15	1	1	0	n/a	1	0	N	Y	Y	Y
mushroom	1 tbsp	14	0	2	0	2	1	0	N	Y	Y	Y
oyster	1 tbsp	5	0	0	1	0	0	0	Y	Y	Y	Y
spaghetti	1/4 c	57	1.5	8	2	0	2	0	N	Δ	Y	Y
stroganoff	1 tbsp	50	2	8	0	0	1	1	N	N	Δ	Y
sweet and sour	1 tbsp	15	0	4	0	3	0	0	N	Δ	Y	Y
taco: red or green	1 tbsp	5-7	0	1	0	0-1	0	0	N	Y	Y	Y
tamari	1 tbsp	10	2	0	0	0	0	0	N	Y	Y	Y
teriyaki	1 tbsp	15	1	3	0	2	0	0	N	Δ	Y	Y
tomato	1/2 c	39	2	9	2	5	0	0	N	Δ	Y	Y
white	1 tbsp	27	1	1	0	0	2	1	N	Δ	Y	Y

FAQ – General

Overall, there is a great deal of commonality among HCG diet protocol information sources, but there are some significant differences of opinion from one source to another source, also. You can find many sites with more HCG FAQ simply by searching HCG FAQ or referencing the websites and forums listed previously in this guide. Remarkably, the manuscript from so many years ago still covers almost all of the frequently asked HCG questions except those relating to new types of HCG applications i.e. sublingual, homeopathic, prescription cream and actual protocol questions including those listed below. Dr. Simeons did his homework indeed.

What is HCG?

HCG (Human Chorionic Gonadotropin) is a hormone naturally produced in large quantity during pregnancy.

Dr. ATW Simeons, the doctor who developed and worked with the protocol for over 15 years, found that small regular doses of HCG caused the body to release abnormal fat when used in conjunction with a specific 500 calorie daily diet. This is detailed in Dr. Simeons' manuscript *Pounds and Inches: A New Approach to Obesity,* which is in the appendix of this book. This low calorie diet is only comfortable and advisable with HCG. Most participants are not hungry and have plenty of energy.

Since this is the 'pregnancy hormone', does it work for men as well? If so, is it safe for men to be putting pregnancy hormone into their bodies?

Yes! The HCG protocol is considered safe for men and even works faster for men. No surprise there, right ladies? While women typically lose .5 lb. – 1lb. per day, men typically lose .75 lb. 2 lbs per day. Since HCG is used in infertility treatment for both men and women by the mainstream medical community, it is considered safe. HCG is also prescribed for men with certain other medical conditions, so this is not the only use of HCG with men.

What are the typical results seen while taking these HCG drops?

We see a typical weight loss of 20-30 lbs in about 30-40 days while following Dr. Simeons' Protocol. This assumes correctly following the low calorie diet and all the other rules (no oily make-up, no lotions, etc.) without cheating or errors.

What are the positive effects of HCG?

Besides the *accelerated weight loss* and *body re-shaping*, many participants report: better, more deep sleep; lower cholesterol and blood pressure while on the HCG, and sometimes continuing afterwards; less insulin or other medications required while on the protocol; higher energy levels without a nervous or edgy feeling; a general feeling of well-being.

What are some negative side effects sometimes experienced while HCG is present in the body?

While on the protocol a few patients report: a headache for the first few days of the protocol (which can be addressed with aspirin, etc.); leg cramping (which can usually be managed with cell salts or other OTC products); temporary hair thinning (the same phenomenon that occurs after child birth or any other weight loss method). Note: There has been significantly less hair loss reported with Homeopathic HCG than injection HCG.

Why the 500 calorie diet (VLCD—very low calorie diet)?

You are on a VLCD (very low calorie diet) of approximately 500 calories because, according to Dr. Simeons, while you are on the HCG, your body is releasing 1500-4000 calories from abnormal fat into your bloodstream each day from your fat reserves. So, theoretically, with the 500 calories you are taking in by mouth plus the 1500-4000 calories being released into your system, you are actually getting the benefit of (500 + 1500-4000) = 2000-4500 calories each day.

What will I eat on this protocol? Do I have to buy your diet food?

Most participants will eat fresh food bought directly from the grocery store. The diet is listed in both the front and back of this book, and is very detailed. There are food options becoming available for convenience such as those listed on www.HCGPerfectPortions.com. As popularity of the HCG Diet grows more resources become available, but many do not follow Dr. Simeons' protocol carefully i.e. companies mix vegetables, use invalid brands of stevia and other sweeteners, etc. So you must be very cautious in finding items. Some products that make the program much more palatable are the Pounds and Inches Away Vinaigrette dressing/marinade, the bouillon, and the seasoning spice which are all made following HCG diet protocol guidelines. There is no mandatory "program food" required to complete the program.

Of course being on a 500 calorie diet will help you to lose weight. How is the HCG protocol different from any other diet out there?

Dr. Simeons, the physician who developed the HCG Protocol, said, "When an obese patient tries to reduce by starving himself, he will first lose his normal fat reserves. When these are exhausted he begins to burn up structural fat, and only as a last resort will the body yield its abnormal reserves, though by that time the patient usually feels so weak and hungry that the diet is abandoned. It is just for this reason that obese patients complain that when they diet they lose the wrong fat. They feel famished and tired and their face becomes drawn and haggard, but their belly, hips, thighs and upper arms show little improvement."

To rephrase Dr. Simeons:
The HCG allows your body to tap into your body's abnormal fat deposits (shoulders, upper arms, belly, hips, thighs, and buttocks). These deposits are not usually accessible to the body until the person has gone through both his normal fat and structural fat as described above. This is the reason why no matter how much some people exercise and starve himself/herself, they still have, for example, a "big butt". The HCG coupled with the very low calorie diet allows a person to tap into abnormal fat deposits which releases nutritious calories into the blood stream to be used by the body. This is similar to how a pregnant woman, who is nauseous for weeks at a time, and not able to keep food down, typically remains healthy and is additionally able to give birth to a healthy baby.

This release of fat/calories into the blood stream is also why clients taking the HCG are generally not hungry and generally have plenty of energy. The HCG actually releases 1500-4000 calories per day into the bloodstream according to Dr. Simeons. By the way, this is the ONLY reason why it is okay to be on a 500 calorie diet. Without the HCG releasing the abnormal fat and, therefore, many calories into the bloodstream, the client would look haggard, be starving, and be facing excessive nutritional deficiency.

Besides tapping into the abnormal fat deposits, HCG also proposes to affect your base metabolism. As yet another positive side effect, this protocol provides a detox and gives your entire system rest from the onslaught of not-so-healthy food and drinks we normally ingest by allowing only a small amount of relatively healthy items to be processed in your body and by your hypothalamus. Some experts feel this 'detox' allows your hypothalamus to clear itself of the chemical build-up that could be preventing weight loss and re-establishes the natural functioning and hormone release of the hypothalamus.

Who developed this protocol? Is it safe?

Dr A.T.W Simeons developed the HCG Protocol in Italy in the 1950's. He worked on the study of obesity for 40 years and on this protocol specifically for about 20 years. He helped countless patients in his clinic. Dr. Simeons found the protocol to be extremely safe and effective.

We concur as we have had hundreds of clients use the protocol with great weight loss and significant improvement in overall health. Keep in mind, this is the same hormone produced *naturally* in a pregnant woman's body. It is also frequently used in infertility treatments for both women and men. Additionally, with infertility and other treatments involving HCG, the HCG administered is substantially higher than the amount administered for weight loss in the HCG Weight Loss Cure Protocol. Just to put it into perspective, Dr. Simeons advised each patient on the HCG protocol to administer **125 units** of HCG per day for a *maximum of 40 days*. However, during pregnancy, a woman can produce up to **1,000,000 units per day**.

Is HCG FDA-Approved?

If you are asking if the FDA has approved HCG for weight loss, the FDA has NOT approved HCG specifically for weight loss. While this may be alarming to some potential participants, we do NOT disagree with the FDA **because** HCG alone does NOT make you lose weight. It is ONLY when HCG is used correctly with Dr. Simeons' HCG Diet Protocol that customers see the amazing typical weight loss of 20-30 lbs in 30-40 days.

Can I continue taking my medications / vitamins while on the HCG Protocol?

For medications, you should always talk to your doctor before stopping or changing any medications. Many participants do just great with medications for high blood pressure, diabetes, high cholesterol, thyroid, and many others. Additionally, if you are on medications, such as for high blood pressure and diabetes, you should be monitored by your physician because some medications require adjustment during the protocol as a natural (and good) side effect of the HCG. However, participants using hormone replacement therapy, steroids, seizure medications, and other medications with "weight gain" as a possible side effect may experience slowed or stalled weight loss.

Regarding the vitamins allowed while on the 500 calorie part of the diet, Dr. Simeons says, "Patients whose teeth are in poor repair sometimes get more trouble under prolonged treatment, just as may occur in pregnancy. In such cases we do allow calcium and vitamin D, though not in an oily solution. The only other vitamin we permit is vitamin C, which we use in large doses combined with an antihistamine at the onset of a common cold. There is no objection to the use of an antibiotic if this is required, for instance by the dentist. In cases of bronchial asthma and hay fever we have occasionally resorted to cortisone during treatment and find that triamcinolone is the least likely to interfere with the loss of weight, but many asthmatics improve with HCG alone".

Is this HCG protocol illegal?

No! While the FDA does not allow anyone to say that HCG causes weight loss, any MD, DO, etc. can write a prescription for the HCG. Use of HCG may be considered 'off label' use of the prescription. This is reasonable since HCG by itself certainly does NOT cause weight loss. More accurately, HCG <u>allows</u> quick, appropriate fat loss when intake is strictly restricted, such as when a pregnant woman cannot eat or keep food down for several days OR when someone is on the 500 calorie phase of the protocol. Many doctors have never heard of Dr. Simeons' protocol and, therefore, may simply choose not to write the prescription due to the FDA's recommendation, but again, physicians are legally able to write the prescription.

Is eating organic required and expensive?

First, it is not required, but recommended because it is healthier for you, but again, not necessary to have successful the weight loss. Second, organic is more expensive, but you can start switching a little at a time as your budget allows. Some estimates for the price difference are 15%, which can probably be afforded on the protocol because you are eating much less food overall.

Is losing weight this fast unhealthy?

Not with the HCG Protocol. Generally, this fast of weight loss would be accompanied by major loss of muscle; however, the HCG makes a huge difference. Participants consistently report losing fat, not muscle, and feeling great.

Isn't skipping breakfast bad for you?

Yes. Except for when you are on the low calorie phase of the HCG protocol because the HCG is releasing the calories from stored fat, so your body is being 'fed' without you taking the calories by mouth.

If I skip breakfast, I feel faint and I have to work, so can I still do it?

For participants who 'need' breakfast, eating ½ of a large apple or a whole piece of fruit (to be taken from the lunch or dinner meal) usually suffices both mentally and physically. We suggest trying the protocol without eating breakfast because many people do just fine while on the HCG. If the 'need' is still there, then go for the fruit or breadsticks from your meals.

Won't I be starving?

Usually…NO! There are some participants who experience some hunger the first 2-5 days of the low calorie diet but even with those participants, the hunger usually disappears after the first week. As a matter of fact, it is not unheard of for participants to report being so 'full' they can't eat all of the food.

Will I gain all the weight back plus some as soon as I stop the 500 calorie phase?

If you perform the maintenance phase correctly and eat like a normal, healthy person, your body should lock-in on your new, lower weight, and maintain your great loss without much effort at all. Review maintenance closely and perform maintenance meticulously to improve your long term future.

Will I need skin removal surgery if I lose 50 or more pounds?

No! Generally, participants are usually quite surprised at the body's ability to reshape to the new body. This is not surprising with HCG since many pregnant women bounce back quite nicely after gaining up to 80 pounds or so during pregnancy. We have monitored clients that have lost over 100 pounds and none have felt the need for surgery. This is just one of the great benefits HCG offers that other diets simply do not.

What makes this protocol different from everything else that's out there?

Dr. Simeons proposed that this wonderful protocol 1) resets the hypothalamus gland so that you go forward with better metabolism to avoid gaining the weight back; 2) reshapes the body by tapping into the abnormal fat such as saddlebags and pear-shaped areas without making the face and chest thin, 3) takes care of the skin as reduction occurs, 4) takes care of hunger, 5) requires no exercise, and 6) usually promotes and overall feeling of well-being.

What about colonics and the specialty teas recommended by Trudeau's book?

Experts disagree on the worthiness of Colonics. Either way, colonics or specialty teas are not required to successfully complete the HCG diet protocol. On the other hand, some specialty teas such as green tea are reported to have health benefits and reduce hunger if hunger is an issue.

I am a busy person, what about eating out?

Most participants are more successful if restaurant eating is avoided. The HCG diet protocol requires a short term commitment, but offers long term results if completed correctly. For emergency purposes, we have found the Mc Donald's grilled chicken breast and side salad with no dressing (or HCG-friendly dressing from www.HCGPerfectPortions.com) is a good, quick backup. Lion's Choice roast beef and celery sticks have also been found to not negatively affect weight loss among many participants. Now if you have to or want to go out for a nice dinner, lobster and asparagus (without butter, of course), shrimp cocktail (no sauce), or small piece of filet are good choices. From our perspective, we can do ANYTHING for 30-40 days especially if the payoff (fat loss) is so significant.

Everyone keeps asking me to explain the diet to them, how do you explain this diet?

If you have friends, family or others asking about the HCG diet protocol and you need help explaining, there is a great video for you to watch at www.PoundsAndInchesAway.com. The video gives a nice brief outline of the protocol to cover the basics.

If any information in this guide was derived, provided as an excerpt, or otherwise displayed from any specific source, the source is prominently given credit along with the information.

The majority of this information was gathered, experienced and divulged by Pounds and Inches Away, Inc. through personal and client experience.

Acknowledgments

Grateful acknowledgement is made to the following authors and HCG advocates:

To Dr. Simeons for decades of research on behalf of the 'Injustice of the Obese'; to Kevin Trudeau for making Dr. Simeons protocol known and available to a new generation through his research and documentation in The Weight Loss Cure "They" Don't Want You To Know About; and to the HCG forums for providing support to individuals who would otherwise simply not be able to experience the weight loss either because of lack of funds, experience, or access.

Appendix: Dr. Simeons' Manuscript

(A couple of changes were made to the following where a typing mistake caused confusion, or a grammatical error made the content hard to follow.)

Pounds & Inches

A NEW APPROACH TO OBESITY

BY: A.T.W. SIMEONS, M.D.

SALVATOR MUNDI INTERNATIONAL HOSPITAL

00152 - ROME

VIALE MURA GIANICOLENSI, 77

FOREWORD

This book discusses a new interpretation of the nature of obesity, and while it does not advocate yet another fancy slimming diet it does describe a method of treatment which has grown out of theoretical considerations based on clinical observation.

What I have to say is, in essence, the views distilled out of forty years of grappling with the fundamental problems of obesity, its causes, its symptoms, and its very nature. In these many years of specialized work, thousands of cases have passed through my hands and were carefully studied. Every new theory, every new method, every promising lead was considered, experimentally screened and critically evaluated as soon as it became known. But invariably the results were disappointing and lacking in uniformity.

I felt that we were merely nibbling at the fringe of a great problem, as, indeed, do most serious students of overweight. We have grown pretty sure that the tendency to accumulate abnormal fat is a very definite metabolic disorder, much as is, for instance, diabetes. Yet the localization and the nature of this disorder remained a mystery. Every new approach seemed to lead into a blind alley, and though patients were told that they are fat because they eat too much, we believed that this is neither the whole truth nor the last word in the matter.

Refusing to be side-tracked by an all too facile interpretation of obesity, I have always held that overeating is the result of the disorder, not its cause, and that we can make little headway until we can build for ourselves some sort of theoretical structure with which to explain the condition. Whether such a structure represents the truth is not important at this moment. What it must do is to give us an intellectually satisfying interpretation of what is happening in the obese body. It must also be able to withstand the onslaught of all hitherto known clinical facts and furnish a hard background against which the results of treatment can be accurately assessed.

To me this requirement seems basic, and it has always been the center of my interest. In dealing with obese patients it became a habit to register and order every clinical experience as if it were an odd looking piece of a jig-saw puzzle. And then, as in a jig saw puzzle, little clusters of fragments began to form, though they seemed to fit in nowhere. As the years passed these clusters grew bigger and started to amalgamate until, about sixteen years ago, a complete picture became dimly discernible. This picture was, and still is, dotted with gaps for which I cannot find the pieces, but I do now feel that a theoretical structure is visible as a whole.

With mounting experience, more and more facts seemed to fit snugly into the new framework, and then, when a treatment based on such speculations showed consistently satisfactory results, I was sure that some practical advance had been made, regardless of whether the theoretical interpretation of these results is correct or not.

The clinical results of the new treatment have been published in scientific journal and these reports have been generally well received by the profession, but the very nature of a scientific article does not permit the full presentation of new theoretical concepts nor is there room to discuss the finer points of technique and the reasons for observing them.

During the 16 years that have elapsed since I first published my findings, I have had many hundreds of inquiries from research institutes, doctors and patients. Hitherto I could only refer those interested to my scientific papers, though I realized that these did not contain sufficient information to enable doctors to conduct the new treatment satisfactorily. Those who tried were obliged to gain their own experience through the many trials and errors which I have long since overcome.

Doctors from all over the world have come to Italy to study the method, first hand in my clinic in the Salvator Mutidi International Hospital in Rome. For some of them the time they could spare has been too short to get a full grasp of the technique, and in any case the number of those whom I have been able to meet personally is small compared with the many requests for further detailed information which keep coming in. I have tried to keep up with these demands by correspondence, but the volume of this work has become unmanageable and that is one excuse for writing this book.

In dealing with a disorder in which the patient must take an active part in the treatment, it is, I believe, essential that he or she have an understanding of what is being done and why. Only then can there be intelligent cooperation between physician and patient. In order to avoid writing two books, one for the physician and another for the patient - a prospect which would probably have resulted in no book at all - I have tried to meet the requirements of both in a single book. This is a rather difficult enterprise in which I may not have succeeded. The expert will grumble about long-windedness while the lay-reader may occasionally have to look up an unfamiliar word in the glossary provided for him.

To make the text more readable I shall be unashamedly authoritative and avoid all the hedging and tentativeness with which it is customarily to express new scientific concepts grown out of clinical experience and not as yet confirmed by clear-cut laboratory experiments. Thus, when I make what reads like a factual statement, the professional reader may have to translate into: clinical experience seems to suggest that such and such an observation might be tentatively explained by such and such a working hypothesis, requiring a vast amount of further research before the hypothesis can be considered a valid theory. If we can from the outset establish this as a mutually accepted convention, I hope to avoid being accused of speculative exuberance.

THE NATURE OF OBESITY

Obesity a Disorder

As a basis for our discussion we postulate that obesity in all its many forms is due to an abnormal functioning of some part of the body and that every ounce of abnormally accumulated fat is always the result of the same disorder of certain regulatory chanisms. Persons suffering from this particular disorder will get fat regardless of whether they eat excessively, normally or less than normal. A person who is free of the disorder will never get fat, even if he frequently overeats.

Those in whom the disorder is severe will accumulate fat very rapidly, those in whom it is moderate will gradually increase in weight and those in whom it is mild may be able to keep their excess weight stationary for long periods. In all these cases a loss of weight brought about by dieting, treatments with thyroid, appetite-reducing drugs, laxatives, violent exercise, massage, or baths is only temporary and will be rapidly regained as soon as the reducing regimen is relaxed. The reason is simply that none of these measures corrects the basic disorder.

While there are great variations in the severity of obesity, we shall consider all the different forms in both sexes and at all ages as always being due to the same disorder. Variations in form would then be partly a matter of degree, partly an inherited bodily constitution and partly the result of a secondary involvement of endocrine glands such as the pituitary, the thyroid, the adrenals or the sex glands. On the other hand, we postulate that no deficiency of any of these glands can ever directly produce the common disorder known as obesity.

If this reasoning is correct, it follows that a treatment aimed at curing the disorder must be equally effective in both sexes, at all ages and in all forms of obesity. Unless this is so, we are entitled to harbor grave doubts as to whether a given treatment corrects the underlying disorder. Moreover, any claim that the disorder has been corrected must be substantiated by the ability of the patient to eat normally of any food he pleases without regaining abnormal fat after treatment. Only if these conditions are fulfilled can we legitimately speak of curing obesity rather than of reducing weight.

Our problem thus presents itself as an enquiry into the localization and the nature of the disorder which leads to obesity. The history of this enquiry is a long series of high hopes and bitter disappointments.

The History of Obesity

There was a time, not so long ago, when obesity was considered a sign of health and prosperity in man and of beauty, amorousness and fecundity in women. This attitude probably dates back to Neolithic times, about 8000 years ago; when for the first time in the history of culture, man began to own property, domestic animals, arable land, houses, pottery and metal tools. Before that, with the possible exception of some races such as the Hottentots, obesity was almost non-existent, as it still is in all wild animals and most primitive races.

Today obesity is extremely common among all civilized races, because a disposition to the disorder can be inherited. Wherever abnormal fat was regarded as an asset, sexual selection tended to propagate the trait. It is only in very recent times that manifest obesity has lost some of its allure, though the cult of the outsize bust - always a sign of latent obesity - shows that the trend still lingers on.

The Significance of Regular Meals

In the early Neolithic times another change took place which may well account for the fact that today nearly all inherited dispositions sooner or later develop into manifest obesity. This change was the institution of regular meals. In pre-Neolithic times, man ate only when he was hungry and only as much as he required too still the pangs of hunger. Moreover, much of his food was raw and all of it was unrefined. He roasted his meat, but he did not boil it, as he had no pots, and what little he may have grubbed from the Earth and picked from the trees, he ate as he went along.

The whole structure of man's omnivorous digestive tract is, like that of an ape, rat or pig, adjusted to the continual nibbling of tidbits. It is not suited to occasional gorging as is, for instance, the intestine of the carnivorous cat family. Thus the institution of regular meals, particularly of food rendered rapidly, placed a great burden on modern man's ability to cope with large quantities of food suddenly pouring into his system from the intestinal tract.

The institution of regular meals meant that man had to eat more than his body required at the moment of eating so as to tide him over until the next meal. Food rendered easily digestible suddenly flooded his body with nourishment of which he was in no need at the moment. Somehow, somewhere this surplus had to be stored.

Three Kinds of Fat

In the human body we can distinguish three kinds of fat. The first is the structural fat which fills the gaps between various organs, a sort of packing material. Structural fat also performs such important functions as bedding the kidneys in soft elastic tissue, protecting the coronary arteries and keeping the skin smooth and taut. It also provides the springy cushion of hard fat under the bones of the feet, without which we would be unable to walk.

The second type of fat is a normal reserve of fuel upon which the body can freely draw when the nutritional income from the intestinal tract is insufficient to meet the demand. Such normal reserves are localized all over the body. Fat is a substance which packs the highest caloric value into the smallest space so that normal reserves of fuel for muscular activity and the maintenance of body temperature can be most economically stored in this form. Both these types of fat, structural and reserve, are normal, and even if the body stocks them to capacity this can never be called obesity.

But there is a third type of fat which is entirely abnormal. It is the accumulation of such fat, and of such fat only, from which the overweight patient suffers. This abnormal fat is also a potential reserve of fuel, but unlike the normal reserves it is not available to the body in a nutritional emergency. It is, so to speak, locked away in a fixed deposit and is not kept in a current account, as are the normal reserves.

When an obese patient tries to reduce by starving himself, he will first lose his normal fat reserves. When these are exhausted he begins to burn up structural fat, and only as a last resort will the body yield its abnormal reserves, though by that time the patient usually feels so weak and hungry that the diet is abandoned. It is just for this reason that obese patients complain that when they diet they lose the wrong fat. They feel famished and tired and their face becomes drawn and haggard, but their belly, hips, thighs and upper arms show little improvement. The fat they have come to detest stays on and the fat they need to cover their bones gets less and less. Their skin wrinkles and they look old and miserable. And that is one of the most frustrating and depressing experiences a human being can have.

Injustice to the Obese

When then obese patients are accused of cheating, gluttony, lack of will power, greed and sexual complexes, the strong become indignant and decide that modern medicine is a fraud and its representatives fools, while the weak just give up the struggle in despair. In either case the result is the same: a further gain in weight, resignation to an abominable fate and the resolution at least to live tolerably the short span allotted to them - a fig for doctors and insurance companies.

Obese patients only feel physically well as long as they are stationary or gaining weight. They may feel guilty, owing to the lethargy and indolence always associated with obesity. They may feel ashamed of what they have been led to believe is a lack of control. They may feel horrified by the appearance of their nude body and the tightness of their clothes. But they have a primitive feeling of animal content which turns to misery and suffering as soon as they make a resolute attempt to reduce. For this there are sound reasons.

In the first place, more caloric energy is required to keep a large body at a certain temperature than to heat a small body. Secondly the muscular effort of moving a heavy body is greater than in the case of a light body. The muscular effort consumes calories which must be provided by food. Thus, all other factors being equal, a fat person requires more food than a lean one. One might therefore reason that if a fat person eats only the additional food his body requires he should be able to keep his weight stationary. Yet every physician who has studied obese patients under rigorously controlled conditions knows that this is not true. Many obese patients actually gain weight on a diet which is calorically deficient for their basic needs. There must thus be some other mechanism at work.

Glandular Theories

At one time it was thought that this mechanism might be concerned with the sex glands. Such a connection was suggested by the fact that many juvenile obese patients show an under-development of the sex organs. The middle-age spread in men and the tendency of many women to put on weight in the menopause seemed to indicate a causal connection between diminishing sex function and overweight. Yet, when highly active sex hormones became available, it was found that their administration had no effect whatsoever on obesity. The sex glands could therefore not be the seat of the disorder.

The Thyroid Gland

When it was discovered that the thyroid gland controls the rate at which body-fuel is consumed, it was thought that by administering thyroid gland to obese patients their abnormal fat deposits could be burned up more rapidly. This too proved to be entirely disappointing, because as we now know, these abnormal deposits take no part in the body's energy-turnover - they are inaccessibly locked away. Thyroid medication merely forces the body to consume its normal fat reserves, which are already depleted in obese patients, and then to break down structurally essential fat without touching the abnormal deposits. In this way a patient may be brought to the brink of starvation in spite of having a hundred pounds of fat to spare. **Thus any weight loss brought about by thyroid medication is always at the expense of fat of which the body is in dire need.**

While the majority of obese patients have a perfectly normal thyroid gland and some even have an overactive thyroid, one also occasionally sees a case with a real thyroid deficiency. In such cases, treatment with thyroid brings about a small loss of weight, but this is not due to the loss of any abnormal fat. It is entirely the result of the elimination of a mucoid substance, called myxedema, which the body accumulates when there is a marked primary thyroid deficiency. Moreover, patients suffering only from a severe lack of thyroid hormone never become obese in the true sense. Possibly also the observation that normal persons - though not the obese - lose weight rapidly when their thyroid becomes overactive may have contributed to the false notion that thyroid deficiency and obesity are connected. Much misunderstanding about the supposed role of the thyroid gland in obesity is still met with, and it is now really high time that thyroid preparations be once and for all struck off the list of remedies for obesity. This is particularly so because giving thyroid gland to an obese patient whose thyroid is either normal or overactive, besides being useless, is decidedly dangerous.

The Pituitary Gland

The next gland to be falsely incriminated was the anterior lobe of the pituitary. This most important gland lies well protected in a bony capsule at the base of the skull. It has a vast number of functions in the body, among which is the regulation of all the other important endocrine glands. The fact that various signs of anterior pituitary deficiency are often associated with obesity raised the hope that the seat of the disorder might be in this gland. But although a large number of pituitary hormones have been isolated and many extracts of the gland prepared, not a single one or any combination of such factors proved to be of any value in the treatment of obesity. Quite recently, however, a fat-mobilizing factor has been found in pituitary glands, but it is still too early to say whether this factor is destined to play a role in the treatment of obesity.

The Adrenals

Recently, a long series of brilliant discoveries concerning the working of the adrenal or suprarenal glands, small bodies which sit atop the kidneys, have created tremendous interest. This interest also turned to the problem of obesity when it was discovered that a condition which in some respects resembles a severe case of obesity - the so called Cushing's Syndrome - was caused by a glandular new-growth of the adrenals or by their excessive stimulation with ACTH, which is the pituitary hormone governing the activity of the outer rind or cortex of the adrenals.

When we learned that an abnormal stimulation of the adrenal cortex could produce signs that resemble true obesity, this knowledge furnished no practical means of treating obesity by decreasing the activity of the adrenal cortex. There is no evidence to suggest that in obesity there is any excess of adrenocortical activity; in fact, all the evidence points to the contrary. There seems to be rather a lack of adrenocortical function and a decrease in the secretion of ACTH from the anterior pituitary lobe.

So here again our search for the mechanism which produces obesity led us into a blind alley. Recently, many students of obesity have reverted to the nihilistic attitude that obesity is caused simply by overeating and that it can only be cured by under eating.

The Diencephalon or Hypothalamus

For those of us who refused to be discouraged there remained one slight hope. Buried deep down in the massive human brain there is a part which we have in common with all vertebrate animals the so-called diencephalon. It is a very primitive part of the brain and has in man been almost smothered by the huge masses of nervous tissue with which we think, reason and voluntarily move our body. The diencephalon is the part from which the central nervous system controls all the automatic animal functions of the body, such as breathing, the heart beat, digestion, sleep, sex, the urinary system, the autonomous or vegetative nervous system and via the pituitary the whole interplay of the endocrine glands.

It was therefore not unreasonable to suppose that the complex operation of storing and issuing fuel to the body might also be controlled by the diencephalon. It has long been known that the content of sugar - another form of fuel - in the blood depends on a certain nervous center in the diencephalon. When this center is destroyed in laboratory animals, they develop a condition rather similar to human stable diabetes. It has also long been known that the destruction of another diencephalic center produces a voracious appetite and a rapid gain in weight in animals which never get fat spontaneously.

The Fat-Bank

Assuming that in man such a center controlling the movement of fat does exist, its function would have to be much like that of a bank. When the body assimilates from the intestinal tract more fuel than it needs at the moment, this surplus is deposited in what may be compared with a current account. Out of this account it can always be withdrawn as required. All normal fat reserves are in such a current account, and it is probable that a diencephalic center manages the deposits and withdrawals.

When now, for reasons which will be discussed later, the deposits grow rapidly while small withdrawals become more frequent, a point may be reached which goes beyond the diencephalon's banking capacity. Just as a banker might suggest to a wealthy client that instead of accumulating a large and unmanageable current account he should invest his surplus capital, the body appears to establish a fixed deposit into which all surplus funds go but from which they can no longer be withdrawn by the procedure used in a current account. In this way the diencephalic "fat-bank" frees itself from all work which goes beyond its normal banking capacity. The onset of obesity dates from the moment the diencephalon adopts this labor-saving ruse. Once a fixed deposit has been established the normal fat reserves are held at a minimum, while every available surplus is locked away in the fixed deposit and is therefore taken out of normal circulation.

Three Basic Causes of Obesity

(1) The Inherited Factor

Assuming that there is a limit to the diencephalon's fat banking capacity, it follows that there are three basic ways in which obesity can become manifest. The first is that the fat-banking capacity is abnormally low from birth. Such a congenitally low diencephalic capacity would then represent the inherited factor in obesity. When this abnormal trait is markedly present, obesity will develop at an early age in spite of normal feeding; this could explain why among brothers and sisters eating the same food at the same table some become obese and others do not.

(2) Other Diencephalic Disorders

The second way in which obesity can become established is the lowering of a previously normal fat-banking capacity owing to some other diencephalic disorder. It seems to be a general rule that when one of the many diencephalic centers is particularly overtaxed; it tries to increase its capacity at the expense of other centers.

In the menopause and after castration the hormones previously produced in the sex-glands no longer circulate in the body. In the presence of normally functioning sex-glands their hormones act as a brake on the secretion of the sex-gland stimulating hormones of the anterior pituitary. When this brake is removed the anterior pituitary enormously increases its output of these sex-gland stimulating hormones, though they are now no longer effective. In the absence of any response from the non-functioning or missing sex glands, there is nothing to stop the anterior pituitary from producing more and more of these hormones. This situation causes an excessive strain on the diencephalic center which controls the function of the anterior pituitary. In order to cope with this additional burden the center appears to draw more and more energy away from other centers, such as those concerned with emotional stability, the blood circulation (hot flushes) and other autonomous nervous regulations, particularly also from the not so vitally important fat-bank.

The so called stable type of diabetes involves the diencephalic blood sugar regulating center the diencephalon tries to meet this abnormal load by switching energy destined for the fat bank over to the sugar-regulating center, with the result that the fat-banking capacity is reduced to the point at which it is forced to establish a fixed deposit and thus initiate the disorder we call obesity. In this case one would have to consider the diabetes the primary cause of the obesity, but it is also possible that the process is reversed in the sense that a deficient or overworked fat-center draws energy from the sugar-center, in which case the obesity would be the cause of that type of diabetes in which the pancreas is not primarily involved. Finally, it is conceivable that in Cushing's syndrome those symptoms which resemble obesity are entirely due to the withdrawal of energy from the diencephalic fat-bank in order to make it available to the highly disturbed center which governs the anterior pituitary adrenocortical system.

Whether obesity is caused by a marked inherited deficiency of the fat-center or by some entirely different diencephalic regulatory disorder, its insurgence obviously has nothing to do with overeating and in either case obesity is certain to develop regardless of dietary restrictions. In these cases any enforced food deficit is made up from essential fat reserves and normal structural fat, much to the disadvantage of the patient's general health.

(3) The Exhaustion of the Fat-bank

But there is still a third way in which obesity can become established, and that is when a presumably normal fat-center is suddenly (with emphasis on suddenly) called upon to deal with an enormous influx of food far in excess of momentary requirements. At first glance it does seem that here we have a straight-forward case of overeating being responsible for obesity, but on further analysis it soon becomes clear that the relation of cause and effect is not so simple. In the first place we are merely assuming that the capacity of the fat center is normal while it is possible and even probable that the only persons who have some inherited trait in this direction can become obese merely by overeating.

Secondly, in many of these cases the amount of food eaten remains the same and it is only the consumption of fuel which is suddenly decreased, as when an athlete is confined to bed for many weeks with a broken bone or when a man leading a highly active life is suddenly tied to his desk in an office and to television at home. Similarly, when a person, grown up in a cold climate, is transferred to a tropical country and continues to eat as before, he may develop obesity because in the heat far less fuel is required to maintain the normal body temperature.

When a person suffers a long period of privation, be it due to chronic illness, poverty, famine or the exigencies of war, his diencephalic regulations adjust themselves to some extent to the low food intake. When then suddenly these conditions change and he is free to eat all the food he wants, this is liable to overwhelm his fat-regulating center. During the WWII about 6000 grossly underfed Polish refugees who had spent harrowing years in Russia were transferred to a camp in India where they were well housed, given normal British army rations and some cash to buy a few extras. Within about three months, 85% were suffering from obesity.

In a person eating coarse and unrefined food, the digestion is slow and only a little nourishment at a time is assimilated from the intestinal tract. When such a person is suddenly able to obtain highly refined foods such as sugar, white flour, butter and oil these are so rapidly digested and assimilated that the rush of incoming fuel which occurs at every meal may eventually overpower the diencephalic regulatory mechanisms and thus lead to obesity. This is commonly seen in the poor man who suddenly becomes rich enough to buy the more expensive refined foods, though his total caloric intake remains the same or is even less than before.

Psychological Aspects

Much has been written about the psychological aspects of obesity. Among its many functions the diencephalon is also the seat of our primitive animal instincts, and just as in an emergency it can switch energy from one center to another, so it seems to be able to transfer pressure from one instinct to another. Thus, a lonely and unhappy person deprived of all emotional comfort and of all instinct gratification except the stilling of hunger and thirst can use these as outlets for pent up instinct pressure and so develop obesity. Yet once that has happened, no amount of psychotherapy or analysis, happiness, company or the gratification of other instincts will correct the condition.

Compulsive Eating

No end of injustice is done to obese patients by accusing them of compulsive eating, which is a form of diverted sex gratification. Most obese patients do not suffer from compulsive eating; they suffer genuine hunger - real, gnawing, torturing hunger - which has nothing whatever to do with compulsive eating. Even their sudden desire for sweets is merely the result of the experience that sweets, pastries and alcohol will most rapidly of all foods allay the pangs of hunger. This has nothing to do with diverted instincts.

On the other hand, compulsive eating does occur in some obese patients, particularly in girls in their late teens or early twenties. Fortunately from the obese patients' greater need for food, it comes on in attacks and is never associated with real hunger, a fact which is readily admitted by the patients. They only feel a feral desire to stuff. Two pounds of chocolates may be devoured in a few minutes; cold, greasy food from the refrigerator, stale bread, leftovers on stacked plates, almost anything edible is crammed down with terrifying speed and ferocity.

I have occasionally been able to watch such an attack without the patient's knowledge, and it is a frightening, ugly spectacle to behold, even if one does realize that mechanisms entirely beyond the patient's control are at work. A careful enquiry into what may have brought on such an attack almost invariably reveals that it is preceded by a strong unresolved sex-stimulation, the higher centers of the brain having blocked primitive diencephalic instinct gratification. The pressure is then let off through another primitive channel, which is oral gratification. In my experience the only thing that will cure this condition is uninhibited sex, a therapeutic procedure which is hardly ever feasible, for if it were, the patient would have adopted it without professional prompting, nor would this in any way correct the associated obesity. It would only raise new and often greater problems if used as a therapeutic measure.

Patients suffering from real compulsive eating are comparatively rare. In my practice they constitute about 1-2%. Treating them for obesity is a heartrending job. They do perfectly well between attacks, but a single bout occurring while under treatment may annul several weeks of therapy. Little wonder that such patients become discouraged. In these cases I have found that psychotherapy may make the patient fully understand the mechanism, but it does nothing to stop it. Perhaps society's growing sexual permissiveness will make compulsive eating even rarer.

Whether a patient is really suffering from compulsive eating or not is hard to decide before treatment because many obese patients think that their desire for food (to them unmotivated) is due to compulsive eating, while all the time it is merely a greater need for food. The only way to find out is to treat such patients. Those that suffer from real compulsive eating continue to have such attacks, while those who are not compulsive eaters never get an attack during treatment.

Reluctance to Lose Weight

Some patients are deeply attached to their fat and cannot bear the thought of losing it. If they are intelligent, popular and successful in spite of their handicap, this is a source of pride. Some fat girls look upon their condition as a safeguard against erotic involvements, of which they are afraid. They work out a pattern of life in which their obesity plays a determining role and then become reluctant to upset this pattern and face a new kind of life which will be entirely different after their figure has become normal and often very attractive. They fear that people will like them - or be jealous - on account of their figure rather than be attracted by their intelligence or character only. Some have a feeling that reducing means giving up an almost cherished and intimate part of them. In many of these cases psychotherapy can be helpful, as it enables these patients to see the whole situation in the full light of consciousness. An affectionate attachment to abnormal fat is usually seen in patients who became obese in childhood, but this is not necessarily so.

In all other cases the best psychotherapy can do in the usual treatment of obesity is to render the burden of hunger and never-ending dietary restrictions slightly more tolerable. Patients who have successfully established an erotic transfer to their psychiatrist are often better able to bear their suffering as a secret labor of love.

There are thus a large number of ways in which obesity can be initiated, though the disorder itself is always due to the same mechanism, an inadequacy of the diencephalic fat-center and the laying down of abnormally fixed fat deposits in abnormal places. This means that once obesity has become established, it can no more be cured by eliminating those factors which brought it on than a fire can be extinguished by removing the cause of the conflagration. Thus a discussion of the various ways in which obesity can become established is useful from a preventative point of view, but it has no bearing on the treatment of the established condition. The elimination of factors which are clearly hastening the course of the disorder may slow down its progress or even halt it, but they can never correct it.

Not by Weight alone

Weight alone is not a satisfactory criterion by which to judge whether a person is suffering from the disorder we call obesity or not. Every physician is familiar with the sylphlike lady who enters the consulting room and declares emphatically that she is getting horribly fat and wishes to reduce. Many an honest and sympathetic physician at once concludes that he is dealing with a "nut." If he is busy he will give her short shrift, but if he has time he will weigh her and show her tables to prove that she is actually underweight.

I have never yet seen or heard of such a lady being convinced by either procedure. The reason is that in my experience the lady is nearly always right and the doctor wrong. When such a patient is carefully examined one finds many signs of potential obesity, which is just about to become manifest as overweight. The patient distinctly feels that something is wrong with her, that a subtle change is taking place in her body, and this alarms her.

There are a number of signs and symptoms which are characteristic of obesity. In manifest obesity many and often all these signs and symptoms are present. In latent or just beginning cases some are always found, and it should be a rule that if two or more of the bodily signs are present, the case must be regarded as one that needs immediate help.

Signs and symptoms of obesity

The bodily signs may be divided into such as have developed before puberty, indicating a strong inherited factor, and those which develop at the onset of manifest disorder. Early signs are a disproportionately large size of the two upper front teeth, the first incisor, or a dimple on both sides of the sacral bone just above the buttocks. When the arms are outstretched with the palms upward, the forearms appear sharply angled outward from the upper arms. The same applies to the lower extremities. The patient cannot bring his feet together without the knees overlapping; he is, in fact, knock-kneed.

The beginning accumulation of abnormal fat shows as a little pad just below the nape of the neck, colloquially known as the Duchess' Hump. There is a triangular fatty bulge in front of the armpit when the arm is held against the body. When the skin is stretched by fat rapidly accumulating under it, it many split in the lower layers. When large and fresh, such tears are purple, but later they are transformed into white scar-tissue. Such striation, as it is called, commonly occurs on the abdomen of women during pregnancy, but in obesity it is frequently found on the breasts, the hips and occasionally on the shoulders. In many cases striation is so fine that the small white lines are only just visible. They are always a sure sign of obesity, and though this may be slight at the time of examination such patients can usually remember a period in their childhood when they were excessively chubby.

Another typical sign is a pad of fat on the insides of the knees, a spot where normal fat reserves are never stored. There may be a fold of skin over the pubic area and another fold may stretch round both sides of the chest, where a loose roll of fat can be picked up between two fingers. In the male an excessive accumulation of fat in the breasts is always indicative, while in the female the breast is usually, but not necessarily, large. Obviously excessive fat on the abdomen, the hips, thighs, upper arms, chin and shoulders are characteristic, and it is important to remember that any number of these signs may be present in persons whose weight is statistically normal; particularly if they are dieting on their own with iron determination.

Common clinical symptoms which are indicative only in their association and in the frame of the whole clinical picture are: frequent headaches, rheumatic pains without detectable bony abnormality; a feeling of laziness and lethargy, often both physical and mental and frequently associated with insomnia, the patients saying that all they want is to rest; the frightening feeling of being famished and sometimes weak with hunger two to three hours after a hearty meal and an irresistible yearning for sweets and starchy food which often overcomes the patient quite suddenly and is sometimes substituted by a desire for alcohol; constipation and a spastic or irritable colon are unusually common among the obese, and so are menstrual disorders.

Returning once more to our sylphlike lady, we can say that a combination of some of these symptoms with a few of the typical bodily signs is sufficient evidence to take her case seriously. A human figure, male or female, can only be judged in the nude; any opinion based on the dressed appearance can be quite fantastically wide off the mark, and I feel myself driven to the conclusion that apart from frankly psychotic patients such as cases of anorexia nervosa; a morbid weight fixation does not exist. I have yet to see a patient who continues to complain after the figure has been rendered normal by adequate treatment.

The Emaciated Lady

I remember the case of a lady who was escorted into my consulting room while I was telephoning. She sat down in front of my desk, and when I looked up to greet her I saw the typical picture of advanced emaciation. Her dry skin hung loosely over the bones of her face, her neck was scrawny and collarbones and ribs stuck out from deep hollows. I immediately thought of cancer and decided to which of my colleagues at the hospital I would refer her. Indeed, I felt a little annoyed that my assistant had not explained to her that her case did not fall under my specialty. In answer to my query as to what I could do for her, she replied that she wanted to reduce. I tried to hide my surprise, but she must have noted a fleeting expression, for she smiled and said "I know that you think I'm mad, but just wait." With that she rose and came round to my side of the desk. Jutting out from a tiny waist she had enormous hips and thighs.

By using a technique which will presently be described, the abnormal fat on her hips was transferred to the rest of her body which had been emaciated by months of very severe dieting. At the end of a treatment lasting five weeks, she, a small woman, had lost 8 inches round her hips, while her face looked fresh and florid, the ribs were no longer visible and her weight was the same to the ounce as it had been at the first consultation.

Fat but not Obese

While a person who is statistically underweight may still be suffering from the disorder which causes obesity, it is also possible for a person to be statistically overweight without suffering from obesity. For such persons weight is no problem, as they can gain or lose at will and experience no difficulty in reducing their caloric intake. They are masters of their weight, which the obese are not. Moreover, their excess fat shows no preference for certain typical regions of the body, as does the fat in all cases of obesity. Thus, the decision whether a borderline case is really suffering from obesity or not cannot be made merely by consulting weight tables.

The Treatment Of Obesity

If obesity is always due to one very specific diencephalic deficiency, it follows that the only way to cure it is to correct this deficiency. At first this seemed an utterly hopeless undertaking. The greatest obstacle was that one could hardly hope to correct an inherited trait localized deep inside the brain, and while we did possess a number of drugs whose point of action was believed to be in the diencephalons, none of them had the slightest effect on the fat-center. There was not even a pointer showing a direction in which pharmacological research could move to find a drug that had such a specific action. The closest approaches were the appetite-reducing drugs - the amphetamines----- but these cured nothing.

A Curious Observation

Mulling over this depressing situation, I remembered a rather curious observation made many years ago in India. At that time we knew very little about the function of the diencephalon, and my interest centered round the pituitary gland. Proehlich had described cases of extreme obesity and sexual underdevelopment in youths suffering from a new growth of the anterior pituitary lobe, producing what then became known as Froehlich's disease. However, it was very soon discovered that the identical syndrome, though running a less fulminating course, was quite common in patients whose pituitary gland was perfectly normal. These are the so-called "fat boys" with long, slender hands, breasts any flat-chested maiden would be proud to posses, large hips, buttocks and thighs with striation, knock-knees and underdeveloped genitals, often with undescended testicles.

It also became known that in these cases the sex organs could he developed by giving the patients injections of a substance extracted from the urine of pregnant women, it having been shown that when this substance was injected into sexually immature rats it made them precociously mature. The amount of substance which produced this effect in one rat was called one International Unit, and the purified extract was accordingly called "Human Chorionic Gonadotrophin" whereby chorionic signifies that it is produced in the placenta and gonadotropin that its action is sex gland directed.

The usual way of treating "fat boys" with underdeveloped genitals is to inject several hundred international Units twice a week. Human Chorionic Gonadotrophin which we shall henceforth simply call HCG is expensive and as "fat boys" are fairly common among Indians I tried to establish the smallest effective dose. In the course of this study three interesting things emerged. The first was that when fresh pregnancy-urine from the female ward was given in quantities of about 300 cc. by retention enema, as good results could be obtained as by injecting the pure substance. The second was that small daily doses appeared to be just as effective as much larger ones given twice a week. Thirdly, and that is the observation that concerns us here, when such patients were given small daily doses they seemed to lose their ravenous appetite though they neither gained nor lost weight. Strangely enough however, their shape did change. Though they were not restricted in diet, there was a distinct decrease in the circumference of their hips.

Fat on the Move

Remembering this, it occurred to me that the change in shape could only be explained by a movement of fat away from abnormal deposits on the hips, and if that were so there was just a chance that while such fat was in transition it might be available to the body as fuel. This was easy to find out, as in that case, fat on the move would be able to replace food. It should then he possible to keep a "fat boy" on a severely restricted diet without a feeling of hunger, in spite of a rapid loss of weight. When I tried this in typical cases of Froehlich's syndrome, I found that as long as such patients were given small daily doses of HCG they could comfortably go about their usual occupations on a diet of only 500 Calories daily and lose an average of about one pound per day. It was also perfectly evident that only abnormal fat was being consumed, as there were no signs of any depletion of normal fat. Their skin remained fresh and turgid, and gradually their figures became entirely normal. The daily administration of HCG appeared to have no side-effects other than beneficial ones.

From this point it was a small step to try the same method in all other forms of obesity. It took a few hundred cases to establish beyond reasonable doubt that the mechanism operates in exactly the same way and seemingly without exception in every case of obesity. I found that, though most patients were treated in the outpatients department, gross dietary errors rarely occurred. On the contrary, most patients complained that the two meals of 250 calories each were more than they could manage, as they continually had a feeling of just having had a large meal.

Pregnancy and Obesity

Once this trail was opened, further observations seemed to fall into line. It is well known that during pregnancy an obese woman can very easily lose weight. She can drastically reduce her diet without feeling hunger or discomfort and lose weight without in any way harming the child in her womb. It is also surprising to what extent a woman can suffer from pregnancy-vomiting without coming to any real harm.

Pregnancy is an obese woman's one great chance to reduce her excess weight. That she so rarely makes use of this opportunity is due to the erroneous notion, usually fostered by her elder relations, that she now has "two mouths to feed" and must "keep up her strength for the coming event. All modern obstetricians know that this is nonsense and that the more superfluous fat is lost the less difficult will be the confinement, though some still hesitate to prescribe a diet sufficiently low in calories to bring about a drastic reduction.

A woman may gain weight during pregnancy, but she never becomes obese in the strict sense of the word. Under the influence of the HCG which circulates in enormous quantities in her body during pregnancy, her diencephalic banking capacity seems to be unlimited, and abnormal fixed deposits are never formed. At confinement she is suddenly deprived of HCG, and her diencephalic fat-center reverts to its normal capacity. It is only then that the abnormally accumulated fat is locked away again in a fixed deposit. From that moment on she is again suffering from obesity and is subject to all its consequences.

Pregnancy seems to be the only normal human condition in which the diencephalic fat banking capacity is unlimited. It is only during pregnancy that fixed fat deposits can be transferred back into the normal current account and freely drawn upon to make up for any nutritional deficit. During pregnancy, every ounce of reserve fat is placed at the disposal of the growing fetus. Were this not so, an obese woman, whose normal reserves are already depleted, would have the greatest difficulties in bringing her pregnancy to full term. There is considerable evidence to suggest that it is the HCG produced in large quantities in the placenta which brings about this diencephalic change.

Though we may be able to increase the diencephalic fat banking capacity by injecting HCG, this does not in itself affect the weight, just as transferring monetary funds from a fixed deposit into a current account does not make a man any poorer; to become poorer it is also necessary that he freely spends the money which thus becomes available. In pregnancy the needs of the growing embryo take care of this to some extent, but in the treatment of obesity there is no embryo, and so a very severe dietary restriction must take its place for the duration of treatment.

Only when the fat which is in transit under the effect of HCG is actually consumed can more fat be withdrawn from the fixed deposits. In pregnancy it would be most undesirable if the fetus were offered ample food only when there is a high influx from the intestinal tract. Ideal nutritional conditions for the fetus can only be achieved when the mother's blood is continually saturated with food, regardless of whether she eats or not, as otherwise a period of starvation might hamper the steady growth of the embryo. It seems that HCG brings about this continual saturation of the blood, which is the reason why obese patients under treatment with HCG never feel hungry in spite of their drastically reduced food intake.

The Nature of Human Chorionic Gonadotropin

HCG is never found in the human body except during pregnancy and in those rare cases in which a residue of placental tissue continues to grow in the womb in what is known as a chorionic epithelioma. It is never found in the male. The human type of chorionic gonadotrophin is found only during the pregnancy of women and the great apes. It is produced in enormous quantities, so that during certain phases of her pregnancy a woman may excrete as much as one million International Units per day in her urine - enough to render a million infantile rats precociously mature. Other mammals make use of a different hormone, which can be extracted from their blood serum but not from their urine. Their placenta differs in this and other respects from that of man and the great apes. This animal chorionic gonadotrophin is much less rapidly broken down in the human body than HCG, and it is also less suitable for the treatment of obesity.

As often happens in medicine, much confusion has been caused by giving HCG its name before its true mode of action was understood. It has been explained that gonadotrophin literally means a sex-gland directed substance or hormone, and this is quite misleading. It dates from the early days when it was first found that HCG is able to render infantile sex glands mature, whereby it was entirely overlooked that it has no stimulating effect whatsoever on normally developed and normally functioning sex-glands. No amount of HCG is ever able to increase a normal sex function. It can only improve an abnormal one and in the young hasten the onset of puberty. However, this is no direct effect. HCG acts exclusively at a diencephalic level and there brings about a considerable increase in the functional capacity of all those centers which are working at maximum capacity.

The Real Gonadotrophins

Two hormones known in the female as follicle stimulating hormone (FSH) and corpus luteum stimulating hormone (LSH) are secreted by the anterior lobe of the pituitary gland. These hormones are real gonadotrophilins because they directly govern the function of the ovaries. The anterior pituitary is in turn governed by the diencephalon, and so when there is an ovarian deficiency the diencephalic center concerned is hard put to correct matters by increasing the secretion from the anterior pituitary of FSH or LSH, as the case may be. When sexual deficiency is clinically present, this is a sign that the diencephalic center concerned is unable, in spite of maximal exertion, to cope with the demand for anterior pituitary stimulation. When then the administration of HCG increases the functional capacity of the diencephalon, all demands can be fully satisfied and the sex deficiency is corrected.

That this is the true mechanism underlying the presumed gonadotrophic action of HCG is confirmed by the fact that when the pituitary gland of infantile rats is removed before they are given HCG, the latter has no effect on their sex-glands. HCG cannot therefore have a direct sex gland stimulating action like that of the anterior pituitary gonadotrophins, as FSH and LSH are justly called. The latter are entirely different substances from that which can be extracted from pregnancy urine and which, unfortunately, is called chorionic gonadotrophin. It would be no more clumsy, and certainly far more appropriate, if HCG were henceforth called chorionic diencephalotrophin.

HCG no Sex Hormone

It cannot he sufficiently emphasized that HCG is not sex-hormone, that its action is identical in men, women, children and in those cases in which the sex-glands no longer function owing to old age or their surgical removal. The only sexual change it can bring about after puberty is an improvement of a pre-existing deficiency. But never stimulation beyond the normal. In an indirect way via the anterior pituitary, HCG regulates menstruation and facilitates conception, but it never virilizes a woman or feminizes a man. It neither makes men grow breasts nor does it interfere with their virility, though where this was deficient it may improve it. It never makes women grow a beard or develop a gruff voice. I have stressed this point only for the sake of my lay readers, because, it is our daily experience that when patients hear the word hormone they immediately jump to the conclusion that this must have something to do with the sex- sphere. They are not accustomed as we are, to think thyroid, insulin, cortisone, adrenalin etc, as hormones.

Importance and Potency of HCG

Owing to the fact that HCG has no direct action on any endocrine gland, its enormous importance in pregnancy has been overlooked and its potency underestimated. Though a pregnant woman can produce as much as one million units per day, we find that the injection of only 125 units per day is ample to reduce weight at the rate of roughly one pound per day, even in a colossus weighing 400 pounds, when associated with a 500-calorie diet. It is no exaggeration to say that the flooding of the female body with HCG is by far the most spectacular hormonal event in pregnancy. It has an enormous protective importance for mother and child, and I even go so far as to say that no woman, and certainly not an obese one, could carry her pregnancy to term without it.

If I can be forgiven for comparing my fellow-endocrinologists with wicked Godmothers, HCG has certainly been their Cinderella, and I can only romantically hope that its extraordinary effect on abnormal fat will prove to be its Fairy Godmother.

HCG has been known for over half a century. It is the substance which Aschheim and Zondek so brilliantly used to diagnose early pregnancy out of the urine. Apart from that, the only thing it did in the experimental laboratory was to produce precocious rats, and that was not particularly stimulating to further research at a time when much more thrilling endocrinological discoveries were pouring in from all sides, sweeping, HCG into the stiller back waters.

Complicating Disorders

Some complicating disorders are often associated with obesity, and these we must briefly discuss. The most important associated disorders and the ones in which obesity seems to play a precipitating or at least an aggravating role are the following: the stable type of diabetes, gout, rheumatism and arthritis, high blood pressure and hardening of the arteries, coronary disease and cerebral hemorrhage.

Apart from the fact that they are often - though not necessarily - associated with obesity, these disorders have two things in common. In all of them, modern research is becoming more and more inclined to believe that diencephalic regulations play a dominant role in their causation. The other common factor is that they either improve or do not occur during pregnancy. In the latter respect they are joined by many other disorders not necessarily associated with obesity. Such disorders are, for instance, colitis, duodenal or gastric ulcers, certain allergies, psoriasis, loss of hair, brittle fingernails, migraine, etc.

If HCG + diet does in the obese bring about those diencephalic changes which are characteristic of pregnancy, one would expect to see an improvement in all these conditions comparable to that seen in real pregnancy. The administration of HCG does in fact do this in a remarkable way.

Diabetes

In an obese patient suffering from a fairly advanced case of stable diabetes of many years duration in which the blood sugar may range from 300-400 mg, it is often possible to stop all anti-diabetes medication after the first few days of treatment. The blood sugar continues to drop from day to day and often reaches normal values in 2-3 weeks. As in pregnancy, this phenomenon is not observed in the brittle type of diabetes, and as some cases that are predominantly stable may have a small brittle factor in their clinical makeup, all obese diabetics have to be kept under a very careful and expert watch.

A brittle case of diabetes is primarily due to the inability of the pancreas to produce sufficient insulin, while in the stable type, diencephalic regulations seem to be of greater importance. That is possibly the reason why the stable form responds so well to the HCG method of treating obesity, whereas the brittle type does not. Obese patients are generally suffering from the stable type, but a stable type may gradually change into a brittle one, which is usually associated with a loss of weight. Thus, when an obese diabetic finds that he is losing weight without diet or treatment, he should at once have his diabetes expertly attended to. There is some evidence to suggest that the change from stable to brittle is more liable to occur in patients who are taking insulin for their stable diabetes.

Rheumatism

All rheumatic pains, even those associated with demonstrable bony lesions, improve subjectively within a few days of treatment, and often require neither cortisone nor salicylates. Again this is a well known phenomenon in pregnancy, and while under treatment with HCG + diet the effect is no less dramatic. As it does not after pregnancy, the pain of deformed joints returns after treatment, but smaller doses of pain-relieving drugs seem able to control it satisfactorily after weight reduction. In any case, the HCG method makes it possible in obese arthritic patients to interrupt prolonged cortisone treatment without a recurrence of pain. This in itself is most welcome, but there is the added advantage that the treatment stimulates the secretion of ACTH in a physiological manner and that this regenerates the adrenal cortex, which is apt to suffer under prolonged cortisone treatment.

Cholesterol

The exact extent to which the blood cholesterol is involved in hardening of the arteries, high blood pressure and coronary disease is not as yet known, but it is now widely admitted that the blood cholesterol level is governed by diencephalic mechanisms. The behavior of circulating cholesterol is therefore of particular interest during the treatment of obesity with HCG. Cholesterol circulates in two forms, which we call free and esterified. Normally these fractions are present in a proportion of about 25% free to 75% esterified cholesterol, and it is the latter fraction which damages the walls of the arteries. In pregnancy this proportion is reversed and it may be taken for granted that arteriosclerosis never gets worse during pregnancy for this very reason.

To my knowledge, the only other condition in which the proportion of free to esterified cholesterol is reversed is during the treatment of obesity with HCG + diet, when exactly the same phenomenon takes place. This seems an important indication of how closely a patient under HCG treatment resembles a pregnant woman in diencephalic behavior.

When the total amount of circulating cholesterol is normal before treatment, this absolute amount is neither significantly increased nor decreased. But when an obese patient with abnormally high cholesterol and already showing signs of arteriosclerosis is treated with HCG, his blood pressure drops and his coronary circulation seems to improve, and yet his total blood cholesterol may soar to heights never before reached.

At first this greatly alarmed us. But when we saw that the patients came to no harm even if treatment was continued and we found the same in follow-up examinations undertaken some months after treatment was continued as we found in examinations undertaken some months before treatment. As the increase is mostly in the form of the not dangerous form of the free cholesterol, we gradually came to welcome the phenomenon. Today we believe that the rise is entirely due to the liberation of recent cholesterol deposits that have not yet undergone calcification in the arterial wall and is therefore highly beneficial.

Gout
An identical behavior is found in the blood uric acid level of patients suffering from gout. Predictably such patients get an acute and often severe attack after the first few days of HCG treatment but then remain entirely free of pain, in spite of the fact that their blood uric acid often shows a marked increase which may persist for several months after treatment. Those patients who have regained their normal weight remain free of symptoms regardless of what they eat, while those that require a second course of treatment get another attack of gout as soon as the second course is initiated. We do not yet know what diencephalic mechanisms are involved in gout; possibly emotional factors play a role, and it is worth remembering that the disease does not occur in women of childbearing age. We now give 2 tablets daily of ZYLORIC to all patients who give a history of gout and have a high blood uric acid level. In this way we can completely avoid attacks during treatment.

Blood Pressure
Patients, who have brought themselves to the brink of malnutrition by exaggerated dieting, laxatives etc, often have an abnormally low blood pressure. In these cases the blood pressure rises to normal values at the beginning of treatment and then very gradually drops, as it always does in patients with a normal blood pressure. Normal values are always regained a few days after the treatment is over. Of this lowering of the blood pressure during treatment the patients are not aware. When the blood pressure is abnormally high, and provided there are no detectable renal lesions, the pressure drops, as it usually does in pregnancy. The drop is often very rapid, so rapid in fact that it sometimes is advisable to slow down the process with pressure sustaining medication until the circulation has had a few days time to adjust itself to the new situation. On the other hand, among the thousands of cases treated, we have never seen any incident which could be attributed to the rather sudden drop in high blood pressure.

When a woman suffering from high blood pressure becomes pregnant her blood pressure very soon drops, but after her confinement it may gradually rise back to its former level. Similarly, a high blood pressure present before HCG treatment tends to rise again after the treatment is over, though this is not always the case. But the former high levels are rarely reached, and we have gathered the impression that such relapses respond better to orthodox drugs such as Reserpine than before treatment.

Peptic Ulcers
In our cases of obesity with gastric or duodenal ulcers we have noticed a surprising subjective improvement in spite of a diet which would generally be considered most inappropriate for an ulcer patient. Here, too, there is a similarity with pregnancy, in which peptic ulcers hardly ever occur. However we have seen two cases with a previous history of several hemorrhages in which a bleeding occurred within 2 weeks of the end of treatment.

Psoriasis, Fingernails, Hair Varicose Ulcers
As in pregnancy, psoriasis greatly improves during treatment but may relapse when the treatment is over. Most patients spontaneously report a marked improvement in the condition of brittle fingernails. The loss of hair not infrequently associated with obesity is temporarily arrested, though in very rare cases an increased loss of hair has been reported. I remember a case in which a patient developed a patchy baldness - so called alopecia areata - after a severe emotional shock, just before she was about to start an HCG treatment. Our dermatologist diagnosed the case as a particularly severe one, predicting that all the hair would be lost. He counseled against the reducing treatment, but in view of my previous experience and as the patient was very anxious not to postpone reducing, I discussed the matter with the dermatologist and it was agreed that, having fully acquainted the patient with the situation, the treatment should be started. During the treatment, which lasted four weeks, the further development of the bald patches was

almost, if not quite, arrested; however, within a week of having finished the course of HCG, all the remaining hair fell out as predicted by the dermatologist. The interesting point is that the treatment was able to postpone this result but not to prevent it. The patient has now grown a new shock of hair of which she is justly proud.

In obese patients with large varicose ulcers we were surprised to find that these ulcers heal rapidly under treatment with HCG. We have since treated non obese patients suffering from varicose ulcers with daily injections of HCG on normal diet with equally good results.

The "Pregnant" Male

When a male patient hears that he is about to be put into a condition which in some respects resembles pregnancy, he is usually shocked and horrified. The physician must therefore carefully explain that this does not mean that he will be feminized and that HCG in no way interferes with his sex. He must be made to understand that in the interest of the propagation of the species nature provides for a perfect functioning of the regulatory headquarters in the diencephalon during pregnancy and that we are merely using this natural safeguard as a means of correcting the diencephalic disorder which is responsible for his overweight.

Technique

Warnings

I must warn the lay reader that what follows is mainly for the treating physician and most certainly not a do-it-yourself primer. Many of the expressions used mean something entirely different to a qualified doctor than that which their common use implies, and only a physician can correctly interpret the symptoms which may arise during treatment. Any patient who thinks he can reduce by taking a few "shots" and eating less is not only sure to be disappointed but may be heading for serious trouble. The benefit the patient can derive from reading this part of the book is a fuller realization of how very important it is for him to follow to the letter his physician's instructions.

In treating obesity with the HCG + diet method we are handling what is perhaps the most complex organ in the human body. The diencephalon's functional equilibrium is delicately poised, so that whatever happens in one part has repercussions in others. In obesity this balance is out of kilter and can only be restored if the technique I am about to describe is followed implicitly. Even seemingly insignificant deviations, particularly those that at first sight seem to be an improvement, are very liable to produce most disappointing results and even annul the effect completely. For instance, if the diet is increased from 500 to 600 or 700 Calories, the loss of weight is quite unsatisfactory. If the daily dose of HCG is raised to 200 or more units daily its action often appears to be reversed, possibly because larger doses evoke diencephalic counter-regulations. On the other hand, the diencephalon is an extremely robust organ in spite of its unbelievable intricacy. From an evolutionary point of view it is one of the oldest organs in our body and its evolutionary history dates back more than 500 million years. This has tendered it extraordinarily adaptable to all natural exigencies, and that is one of the main reasons why the human species was able to evolve. What its evolution did not prepare it for were the conditions to which human culture and civilization now expose it.

History taking

When a patient first presents himself for treatment, we take a general history and note the time when the first signs of overweight were observed. We try to establish the highest weight the patient has ever had in his life (obviously excluding pregnancy), when this was, and what measures have hitherto been taken in an effort to reduce.

It has been our experience that those patients who have been taking thyroid preparations for long periods have a slightly lower average loss of weight under treatment with HCG than those who have never taken thyroid. This is even so in those patients who have been taking thyroid because they had an abnormally low basal metabolic rate. In many of these cases the low BMR is not due to any intrinsic deficiency of the thyroid gland, but rather to a lack of diencephalic stimulation of the thyroid gland via the anterior pituitary lobe. We never allow thyroid to be taken during treatment, and yet a BMR which was very low before treatment is usually found to be normal after a week or two of HCG + diet. Needless to say, this does not apply to those cases in which a thyroid deficiency has been produced by the surgical removal of a part of an overactive gland. It is also most important to ascertain whether the patient has taken diuretics (water eliminating pills) as this also decreases the weight loss under the HCG regimen.

Returning to our procedure, we next ask the patient a few questions to which he is held to reply simply with "yes" or "no". These questions are: Do you suffer from headaches? rheumatic pains? menstrual disorders? constipation? breathlessness or exertion? swollen ankles? Do you consider yourself greedy? Do you feel the need to eat snacks between meals?

The patient then strips and is weighed and measured. The normal weight for his height, age, skeletal and muscular build is established from tables of statistical averages, whereby in women it is often necessary to make an allowance for particularly large and heavy breasts. The degree of overweight is then calculated, and from this the duration of treatment can be roughly assessed on the basis of an average loss of weight of a little less than a pound, say 300-400 grams-per injection, per day. It is a particularly interesting feature of the HCG treatment that in reasonably cooperative patients this figure is remarkably constant, regardless of sex, age and degree of overweight.

The Duration of Treatment

Patients who need to lose 15 pounds (7 kg.) or less require 26 days treatment with 23 daily injections. The extra three days are needed because all patients must continue the 500-calorie diet for three days after the last injection. This is a very essential part of the treatment, because if they start eating normally as long as there is even a trace of HCG in their body they put on weight alarmingly at the end of the treatment. After three days when all the HCG has been eliminated this does not happen, because the blood is then no longer saturated with food and can thus accommodate an extra influx from the intestines without increasing its volume by retaining water.

We never give a treatment lasting less than 26 days, even in patients needing to lose only 5 pounds. It seems that even in the mildest cases of obesity the diencephalon requires about three weeks rest from the maximal exertion to which it has been previously subjected in order to regain fully its normal fat-banking capacity. Clinically this expresses itself, in the fact that, when in these mild cases, treatment is stopped as soon as the weight is normal, which may be achieved in a week, it is much more easily regained than after a full course of 23 injections.

As soon as such patients have lost all their abnormal superfluous fat, they at once begin to feel ravenously hungry with continued injections. This is because HCG only puts abnormal fat into circulation and cannot, in the doses used, liberate normal fat deposits; indeed, it seems to prevent their consumption. As soon as their statistically normal weight is reached, these patients are put on 800-1000 calories for the rest of the treatment. The diet is arranged in such a way that the weight remains perfectly stationary and is thus continued for three days after the 23rd injection. Only then are the patients free to eat anything they please except sugar and starches for the next three weeks.

Such early cases are common among actresses, models, and persons who are tired of obesity, having seen its ravages in other members of their family. Film actresses frequently explain that they must weigh less than normal. With this request we flatly refuse to comply, first, because we undertake to cure a disorder, not to create a new one, and second, because it is in the nature of the HCG method that it is self limiting. It becomes completely ineffective as soon as all abnormal fat is consumed. Actresses with a slight tendency to obesity, having tried all manner of reducing methods, invariably come to the conclusion that their figure is satisfactory only when they are underweight, simply because none of these methods remove their superfluous fat deposits. When they see that under HCG their figure improves out of all proportion to the amount of weight lost, they are nearly always content to remain within their normal weight-range.

When a patient has more than 15 pounds to lose the treatment takes longer but the maximum we give in a single course is 40 injections, nor do we as a rule allow patients to lose more than 34 lbs. (15 Kg.) at a time. The treatment is stopped when either 34 lbs. have been lost or 40 injections have been given. **The only exception we make is in the case of grotesquely obese patients who may be allowed to lose an additional 5-6 lbs. if this occurs before the 40 injections are up.**

Immunity to HCG

The reason for limiting a course to 40 injections is that by then some patients may begin to show signs of HCG immunity. Though this phenomenon is well known, we cannot as yet define the underlying mechanism. Maybe after a certain length of time the body learns to break down and eliminate HCG very rapidly, or possibly prolonged treatment leads to some sort of counter-regulation which annuls the diencephalic effect.

After 40 daily injections it takes about six weeks before this so called immunity is lost and HCG again becomes fully effective. Usually after about 40 injections patients may feel the onset of immunity as hunger which was previously absent. In those comparatively rare cases in which signs of immunity develop before the full course of 40 injections has been completed-say at the 35th injection- treatment must be stopped at once, because if it is continued the patients begin to look weary and drawn, feel weak and hungry and any further loss of weight achieved is then always at the expense of normal fat. This is not only undesirable, but normal fat is also instantly regained as soon as the patient is returned to a free diet.

Patients who need only 23 injections may be injected daily, including Sundays, as they never develop immunity. In those that take 40 injections the onset of immunity can be delayed if they are given only six injections a week, leaving out Sundays or any other day they choose, provided that it is always the same day. On the days on which they do not receive the injections they usually feel a slight sensation of hunger. At first we thought that this might be purely psychological, but we found that when normal saline is injected without the patient's knowledge the same phenomenon occurs.

Menstruation

During menstruation no injections are given, but the diet is continued and causes no hardship; yet as soon as the menstruation is over, the patients become extremely hungry unless the injections are resumed at once. It is very impressive to see the suffering of a woman who has continued her diet for a day or two beyond the end of the period without coming for her injection and then to hear the next day that all hunger ceased within a few hours after the injection and to see her once again content, florid and cheerful. While on the question of menstruation it must he added that in teenaged girls the period may in some rare cases be delayed and exceptionally stop altogether. If then later this is artificially induced some weight may be regained.

Further Courses

Patients requiring the loss of more than 34 lbs. must have a second or even more courses. A second course can be started after an interval of not less than six weeks, though the pause can be more than six weeks. When a third, fourth or even fifth course is necessary, the interval between courses should be made progressively longer. Between a second and third course eight weeks should elapse, between a third and fourth course twelve weeks, between a fourth and fifth course twenty weeks and between a fifth and sixth course six months. In this way it is possible to bring about a weight reduction of 100 lbs. and more if required without the least hardship to the patient.

In general, men do slightly better than women and often reach a somewhat higher average daily loss. Very advanced cases do a little better than early ones, but it is a remarkable fact that this difference is only just statistically significant.

Conditions that must be accepted before treatment

On the basis of these data the probable duration of treatment can he calculated with considerable accuracy, and this is explained to the patient. It is made clear to him that during the course of treatment he must attend the clinic daily to be weighed, injected and generally checked. All patients that live in Rome or have resident friends or relations with whom they can stay are treated as out-patients, but patients coming from abroad must stay in the hospital, as no hotel or restaurant can be relied upon to prepare the diet with sufficient accuracy. These patients have their meals, sleep, and attend the clinic in the hospital, but are otherwise free to spend their time as they please in the city and its surroundings sightseeing, sun-bathing or theater-going.

It is also made clear that between courses the patient gets no treatment and is free to eat anything he pleases except starches and sugar during the first 3 weeks. It is impressed upon him that he will have to follow the prescribed diet to the letter and that after the first three days this will cost him no effort, as he will feel no hunger and may indeed have difficulty in getting down the 500 Calories which he will be given. If these conditions are not acceptable the case is refused, as any compromise or half measure is bound to prove utterly disappointing to patient and physician alike and is a waste of time and energy.

Though a patient can only consider himself really cured when he has been reduced to his statistically normal weight, we do not insist that he commit himself to that extent. Even a partial loss of overweight is highly beneficial, and it is our experience that once a patient has completed a first course he is so enthusiastic about the ease with which the - to him surprising - results are achieved that he almost invariably comes back for more. There certainly can be no doubt that in my clinic more time is spent on damping over-enthusiasm than on insisting that the rules of the treatment be observed.

Examining the patient

Only when agreement is reached on the points so far discussed do we proceed with the examination of the patient. A note is made of the size of the first upper incisor, of a pad of fat on the nape of the neck, at the axilla and on the inside of the knees. The presence of striation, a suprapubic fold, a thoracic fold, angulation of elbow and knee joint, breast-development in men and women, edema of the ankles and the state of genital development in the male are noted.

Wherever this seems indicated we X-ray the sella turcica, as the bony capsule which contains the pituitary gland is called, measure the basal metabolic rate, X-ray the chest and take an electrocardiogram. We do a blood-count and a sedimentation rate and estimate uric acid, cholesterol, iodine and sugar in the fasting blood.

Gain before Loss

Patients whose general condition is low, owing to excessive previous dieting, must eat to capacity for about one week before starting treatment, regardless of how much weight they may gain in the process. One cannot keep a patient comfortably on 500 Calories unless his normal fat reserves are reasonably well stocked. It is for this reason also that every case, even those that are actually gaining must eat to capacity of the most fattening food they can get down until they have had the third injection. It is a fundamental mistake to put a patient on 500 Calories as soon as the injections are started, as it seems to take about three injections before abnormally deposited fat begins to circulate and thus become available.

We distinguish between the first three injections, which we call "non-effective" as far as the loss of weight is concerned, and the subsequent injections given while the patient is dieting, which we call "effective". The average loss of weight is calculated on the number of effective injections and from the weight reached on the day of the third injection which may be well above what it was two days earlier when the first injection was given.

Most patients who have been struggling with diets for years and know how rapidly they gain if they let themselves go are very hard to convince of the absolute necessity of gorging for at least two days, and yet this must he insisted upon categorically if the further course of treatment is to run smoothly. Those patients who have to be put on forced feeding for a week before starting the injections usually gain weight rapidly - four to six pounds in 24 hours is not unusual - but after a day or two this rapid gain generally levels off. In any case, the whole gain is usually lost in the first 48 hours of dieting. It is necessary to proceed in this manner because the gain re-stocks the depleted normal reserves, whereas the subsequent loss is from the abnormal deposits only.

Patients in a satisfactory general condition and those who have not just previously restricted their diet start forced feeding on the day of the first injection. Some patents say that they can no longer overeat because their stomach has shrunk after years of restrictions. While we know that no stomach ever shrinks, we compromise by insisting that they eat frequently of highly concentrated foods such as milk chocolate, pastries with whipped cream sugar, fried meats (particularly pork), eggs and bacon, mayonnaise, bread with thick butter and jam, etc. The time and trouble spent on pressing this point upon incredulous or reluctant patients is always amply rewarded afterwards by the complete absence of those difficulties which patients who have disregarded these instructions are liable to experience.

During the two days of forced feeding from the first to the third injection - many patients are surprised that contrary to their previous experience they do not gain weight and some even lose. The explanation is that in these cases there is a compensatory flow of urine, which drains excessive water from the body. To some extent this seems to be a direct action of HCG, but it may also be due to a higher protein intake, as we know that a protein-deficient diet makes the body retain water.

Starting treatment

In menstruating women, the best time to start treatment is immediately after a period. Treatment may also be started later, but it is advisable to have at least ten days in hand before the onset of the next period. Similarly, the end of a course should never be made to coincide with onset of menstruation. If things should happen to work out that way, it is better to give the last injection three days before the expected date of the menses so that a normal diet can he resumed at onset. Alternatively, at least three injections should be given after the period, followed by the usual three days of dieting. This rule need not be observed in such patients who have reached their normal weight before the end of treatment and are already on a higher caloric diet.

Patients who require more than the minimum of 23 injections and who therefore skip one day a week in order to postpone immunity to HCG cannot have their third injections on the day before the interval. Thus if it is decided to skip Sundays, the treatment can be started on any day of the week except Thursdays. Supposing they start on Thursday, they will have their third injection on Saturday, which is also the day on which they start their 500 Calorie diet. They would then base no injection on the second day of dieting; this exposes them to an unnecessary hardship, as without the injection they will feel particularly hungry. Of course, the difficulty can be overcome by exceptionally injecting them on the first Sunday. If this day falls between the first and second or between the second and third injection, we usually prefer to give the patient the extra day of forced feeding, which the majority rapturously enjoy.

The Diet

The 500 calorie diet is explained on the day of the second injection to those patients who will be preparing their own food, and it is most important that the person who will actually cook is present - the wife, the mother or the cook, as the case may be. Here in Italy patients are given the following diet sheet.

Breakfast: Tea or coffee in any quantity without sugar. Only one tablespoonful of milk allowed in 24 hours. Saccharin or Stevia may be used.

Lunch:

1. 100 grams of veal, beef, chicken breast, fresh white fish, lobster, crab, or shrimp. All visible fat must be carefully removed before cooking, and the meat must be weighed raw. It must be boiled or grilled without additional fat. Salmon, eel, tuna, herring, dried or pickled fish are not allowed. The chicken breast must be removed from the bird.

2. One type of vegetable only to be chosen from the following: spinach, chard, chicory, beet-greens, green salad, tomatoes, celery, fennel, onions, red radishes, cucumbers, asparagus, cabbage.

3. One breadstick (grissino) or one Melba toast.

4. An apple or a handful of strawberries or one-half grapefruit or orange.

Dinner : The same four choices as lunch.

The juice of one lemon daily is allowed for all purposes. Salt, pepper, vinegar, mustard powder, garlic, sweet basil, parsley, thyme, marjoram, etc., may be used for seasoning, but no oil, butter or dressing.

Tea, coffee, plain water, or mineral water are the only drinks allowed, but they may be taken in any quantity and at all times.

In fact, the patient should drink about 2 liters of these fluids per day. Many patients are afraid to drink so much because they fear that this may make them retain more water. This is a wrong notion as the body is more inclined to store water when the intake falls below its normal requirements.

The fruit or the breadstick may be eaten between meals instead of with lunch or dinner, but not more than four items listed for lunch and dinner may be eaten at one meal.

No medicines or cosmetics other than lipstick, eyebrow pencil and powder may he used without special permission

Every item in the list is gone over carefully, continually stressing the point that no variations other than those listed may be introduced. All things not listed are forbidden, and the patient is assured that nothing permissible has been left out. The 100 grams of meat must he scrupulously weighed raw after all visible fat has been removed. To do this accurately the patient must have a letter-scale, as kitchen scales are not sufficiently accurate and the butcher should certainly not be relied upon. Those not uncommon patients, who feel that even so little food is too much for them, can omit anything they wish.

There is no objection to breaking up the two meals. For instance having a breadstick and an apple for breakfast or before going to bed, provided they are deducted from the regular meals. The whole daily ration of two breadsticks or two fruits may not be eaten at the same time, nor can any item saved from the previous day be added on the following day. In the beginning patients are advised to check every meal against their diet sheet before starting to eat and not to rely on their memory. It is also worth pointing out that any attempt to observe this diet without HCG will lead to trouble in two to three days. We have had cases in which patients have proudly flaunted their dieting powers in front of their friends without mentioning the fact that they are also receiving treatment with HCG. They let their friends try the same diet, and when this proves to be a failure - as it necessarily must - the patient starts raking in unmerited kudos for superhuman willpower.

It should also be mentioned that two small apples weighing as much as one large one never the less have a higher caloric value and are therefore not allowed though there is no restriction on the size of one apple. Some people do not realize that chicken breast does not mean the breast of any other fowl, nor does it mean a wing or drumstick.

The most tiresome patients are those who start counting calories and then come up with all manner of ingenious variations which they compile from their little books. When one has spent years of weary research trying to make a diet as attractive as possible without jeopardizing the loss of weight, culinary geniuses who are out to improve their unhappy lot are hard to take.

Making up the Calories

The diet used in conjunction with HCG must not exceed 500 calories per day, and the way these calories are made up is of utmost importance. For instance, if a patient drops the apple and eats an extra breadstick instead, he will not be getting more calories but he will not lose weight. There are a number of foods, particularly fruits and vegetables, which have the same or even lower caloric values than those listed as permissible, and yet we find that they interfere with the regular loss of weight under HCG, presumably owing to the nature of their composition. Pimiento peppers, okra, artichokes and pears are examples of this.

While this diet works satisfactorily in Italy, certain modifications have to be made in other countries. **For instance, American beef has almost double the caloric value of South Italian beef, which is not marbled with fat. This marbling is impossible to remove**. In America, therefore, low-grade veal should be used for one meal and fish (excluding all those species such as herring, mackerel, tuna, salmon, eel, etc., which have a high fat content, and all dried, smoked or pickled fish), chicken breast, lobster, crawfish, prawns or shrimp, crabmeat or kidneys for the other meal. Where the Italian breadsticks, the so-called grissini, are not available, one Melba toast may be used instead, though they are psychologically less satisfying. A Melba toast has about the same weight as the very porous grissini which is much more to look at and to chew.

When local conditions or the feeding habits of the population make changes necessary it must be borne in mind that the total daily intake must not exceed 500 calories if the best possible results are to be obtained, that the daily ration should contain 200 grams of fat-free protein and a very small amount of starch.

Just as the daily dose of HCG is the same in all cases, so the same diet proves to be satisfactory for a small elderly lady of leisure or a hard working muscular giant. Under the effect of HCG the obese body is always able to obtain all the calories it needs from the abnormal fat deposits, regardless of whether it uses up 1500 or 4000 per day. It must be made very clear to the patient that he is living to a far greater extent on the fat which he is losing than on what he eats.

Many patients ask why eggs are not allowed. The contents of two good sized eggs are roughly equivalent to 100 grams of meat, but unfortunately the yolk contains a large amount of fat, which is undesirable. Very occasionally we allow egg - boiled, poached or raw - to patients who develop an aversion to meat, but in this case they must add the white of three eggs to the one they eat whole. In countries where cottage cheese made from skimmed milk is available 100 grams may occasionally be used instead of the meat, but no other cheeses are allowed.

Vegetarians

Strict vegetarians such as orthodox Hindus present a special problem, because milk and curds are the only animal protein they will eat. To supply them with sufficient protein of animal origin they must drink 500 cc. of skimmed milk per day, though part of this ration can be taken as curds. As far as fruit, vegetables and starch are concerned, their diet is the same as that of non-vegetarians; they cannot be allowed their usual intake of vegetable proteins from leguminous plants such as beans or from wheat or nuts, nor can they have their customary rice. In spite of these severe restrictions, their average loss is about half that of non-vegetarians, presumably owing to the sugar content of the milk.

Faulty Dieting

Few patients will take one's word for it that the slightest deviation from the diet has under HCG disastrous results as far as the weight is concerned. This extreme sensitivity has the advantage that the smallest error is immediately detectable at the daily weighing but most patients have to make the experience before they will believe it.

Persons in high official positions such as embassy personnel, politicians, senior executives, etc., who are obliged to attend social functions to which they cannot bring their meager meal must be told beforehand that an official dinner will cost them the loss of about three days treatment, however careful they are and in spite of a friendly and would-be cooperative host. We generally advise them to avoid all around embarrassment, the almost inevitable turn of conversation to their weight problem and the outpouring of lay counsel from their table partners by not letting it be known that they are under treatment. They should take dainty servings of everything, bide what they can under the cutlery and book the gain which may take three days to get rid of as one of the sacrifices which their profession entails. Allowing three days for their correction, such incidents do not jeopardize the treatment, provided they do not occur all too frequently in which case treatment should be postponed to a socially more peaceful season.

Vitamins and anemia

Sooner or later most patients express a fear that they may be running out of vitamins or that the restricted diet may make them anemic. On this score the physician can confidently relieve their apprehension by explaining that every time they lose a pound of fatty tissue, which they do almost daily, only the actual fat is burned up; all the vitamins, the proteins, the blood, and the minerals which this tissue contains in abundance are fed back into the body. Actually, a low blood count not due to any serious disorder of the blood forming tissues improves during treatment, and we have never encountered a significant protein deficiency nor signs of a lack of vitamins in patients who are dieting regularly.

The First Days of Treatment

On the day of the third injection it is almost routine to hear two remarks. One is: "You know, Doctor, I'm sure it's only psychological, but I already feel quite different". So common is this remark, even from very skeptical patients that we hesitate to accept the psychological interpretation. The other typical remark is: "Now that I have been allowed to eat anything I want, I can't get it down. Since yesterday I feel like a stuffed pig. Food just doesn't seem to interest me any more, and I am longing to get on with your diet". Many patients notice that they are passing more urine and that the swelling in their ankles is less even before they start dieting.

On the day of the fourth injection most patients declare that they are feeling fine. They have usually lost two pounds or more, some say they feel a bit empty but hasten to explain that this does not amount to hunger. Some complain of a mild headache of which they have been forewarned and for which they have been given permission to take aspirin.

During the second and third day of dieting - that is, the fifth and sixth injection-these minor complaints improve while the weight continues to drop at about double the usually overall average of almost one pound per day, so that a moderately severe case may by the fourth day of dieting have lost as much as 8- 10 lbs.

It is usually at this point that a difference appears between those patients who have literally eaten to capacity during the first two days of treatment and those who have not. The former feel remarkably well; they have no hunger, nor do they feel tempted when others eat normally at the same table. They feel lighter, more clear-headed and notice a desire to move quite contrary to their previous lethargy. Those who have disregarded the advice to eat to capacity continue to have minor discomforts and do not have the same euphoric sense of self-being until about a week later. It seems that their normal fat reserves require that much more time before they are fully stocked.

Fluctuations in weight loss

After the fourth or fifth day of dieting the daily loss of weight begins to decrease to one pound or somewhat less per day, and there is a smaller urinary output. Men often continue to lose regularly at that rate, but women are more irregular in spite of faultless dieting. There may be no drop at all for two or three days and then a sudden loss which reestablishes the normal average. These fluctuations are entirely due to variations in the retention and elimination of water, which are more marked in women than in men.

The weight registered by the scale is determined by two processes not necessarily synchronized under the influence of HCG. Fat is being extracted from the cells, in which it is stored in the fatty tissue. When these cells are empty and therefore serve no purpose, the body breaks down the cellular structure and absorbs it, but breaking up of useless cells, connective tissue, blood vessels, etc., may lag behind the process of fat-extraction. When this happens the body appears to replace some of the extracted fat with water which is retained for this purpose. As water is heavier than fat the scales may show no loss of weight, although sufficient fat has actually been consumed to make up for the deficit in the 500-Calorie diet. When such tissue is finally broken down, the water is liberated and there is a sudden flood of urine and a marked loss of weight. This simple interpretation of what is really an extremely complex mechanism is the one we give those patients who want to know why it is that on certain days they do not lose, though they have committed no dietary error.

Patients, who have previously regularly used diuretics as a method of reducing, lose fat during the first two or three weeks of treatment which shows in their measurements, but the scale may show little or no loss because they are replacing the normal water content of their body which has been dehydrated. Diuretics should never be used for reducing.

Interruptions of Weight Loss

We distinguish four types of interruption in the regular daily loss. The first is the one that has already been mentioned in which the weight stays stationary for a day or two, and this occurs, particularly towards the end of a course, in almost every case.

The Plateau

The second type of interruption we call a "plateau". A plateau lasts 4-6 days and frequently occurs during the second half of a full course, particularly in patients that have been doing well and whose overall average of nearly a pound per effective injection has been maintained. Those who are losing more than the average all have a plateau sooner or later. A plateau always corrects, itself, but many patients who have become accustomed to a regular daily loss get unnecessarily worried. No amount of explanation convinces them that a plateau does not mean that they are no longer responding normally to treatment.

In such cases we consider it permissible, for purely psychological reasons, to break up the plateau. This can be done in two ways. One is a so-called "apple day". An apple-day begins at lunch and continues until just before lunch of the following day. The patients are given six large apples and are told to eat one whenever they feel the desire though six apples is the maximum allowed. During an apple-day no other food or liquids except plain water are allowed and of water they may only drink just enough to quench an uncomfortable thirst if eating an apple still leaves them thirsty. Most patients feel no need for water and are quite happy with their six apples. Needless to say, an apple-day may never be given on the day on which there is no injection. The apple-day produces a gratifying loss of weight on the following day, chiefly due to the elimination of water. This water is not regained when the patients resume their normal 500-calorie diet at lunch, and on the following days they continue to lose weight satisfactorily.

The other way to break up a plateau is by giving a non-mercurial diuretic for one day. This is simpler for the patient but we prefer the apple-day as we sometimes find that though the diuretic is very effective on the following day it may take two to three days before the normal daily reduction is resumed, throwing the patient into a new fit of despair. It is useless to give either an apple-day or a diuretic unless the weight has been stationary for at least four days without any dietary error having been committed.

Reaching a Former Level

The third type of interruption in the regular loss of weight may last much longer - ten days to two weeks. Fortunately, it is rare and only occurs in very advanced cases, and then hardly ever during the first course of treatment. It is seen only in those patients who during some period of their lives have maintained a certain fixed degree of obesity for ten years or more and have then at some time rapidly increased beyond that weight. When then in the course of treatment the former level is reached, it may take two weeks of no loss, in spite of HCG and diet, before further reduction is normally resumed.

Menstrual Interruption

The fourth type of interruption is the one which often occurs a few days before and during the menstrual period and in some women at the time of ovulation. It must also be mentioned that when a woman becomes pregnant during treatment - and this is by no means uncommon - she at once ceases to lose weight. An unexplained arrest of reduction has on several occasions raised our suspicion before the first period was missed. If in such cases, menstruation is delayed, we stop injecting and do a precipitation test five days later. No pregnancy test should be carried out earlier than five days after the last injection, as otherwise the HCG may give a false positive result.

Oral contraceptives may be used during treatment.

Dietary Errors

Any interruption of the normal loss of weight which does not fit perfectly into one of those categories is always due to some possibly very minor dietary error. Similarly, any gain of more than 100 grams is invariably the result of some transgression or mistake, unless it happens on or about the day of ovulation or during the three days preceding the onset of menstruation, in which case it is ignored. In all other cases the reason for the gain must be established at once.

The patient who frankly admits that he has stepped out of his regimen when told that something has gone wrong is no problem. He is always surprised at being found out, because unless he has seen this himself he will not believe that a salted almond, a couple of potato chips, a glass of tomato juice or an extra orange will bring about a definite increase in his weight on the following day.

Very often he wants to know why extra food weighing one ounce should increase his weight by six ounces. We explain this in the following way: Under the influence of HCG the blood is saturated with food and the blood volume has adapted itself so that it can only just accommodate the 500 calories which come in from the intestinal tract in the course of the day. Any additional income, however little this may be, cannot be accommodated and the blood is therefore forced to increase its volume sufficiently to hold the extra food, which it can only do in a very diluted form. Thus it is not the weight of what is eaten that plays the determining role but rather the amount of water which the body must retain to accommodate this food.

This can be illustrated by mentioning the case of salt. In order to hold one teaspoonful of salt the body requires one liter of water, as it cannot accommodate salt in any higher concentration. Thus, if a person eats one teaspoonful of salt his weight will go up by more than two pounds as soon as this salt is absorbed from his intestine.

To this explanation many patients reply: Well, if I put on that much every time I eat a little extra, how can I hold my weight after the treatment? It must therefore be made clear that this only happens as long as they are under HCG. When treatment is over, the blood is no longer saturated and can easily accommodate extra food without having to increase its volume. Here again the professional reader will be aware that this interpretation is a simplification of an extremely intricate physiological process which actually accounts for the phenomenon.

Salt and Reducing

While we are on the subject of salt, I can take this opportunity to explain that we make no restriction in the use of salt and insist that the patients drink large quantities of water throughout the treatment. We are out to reduce abnormal fat and are not in the least interested in such illusory weight losses as can be achieved by depriving the body of salt and by desiccating it. Though we allow the free use of salt, the daily amount taken should be roughly the same, as a sudden increase will of course be followed by a corresponding increase in weight as shown by the scale. An increase in the intake of salt is one of the most common causes for an increase in weight from one day to the next. Such an increase can be ignored, provided it is accounted for, it in no way influences the regular loss of fat.

Water

Patients are usually hard to convince that the amount of water they retain has nothing to do with the amount of water they drink. When the body is forced to retain water, it will do this at all costs. If the fluid intake is insufficient to provide all the water required, the body withholds water from the kidneys and the urine becomes scanty and highly concentrated, imposing a certain strain on the kidneys. If that is insufficient, excessive water will be with-drawn from the intestinal tract, with the result that the feces become hard and dry. On the other hand if a patient drinks more than his body requires, the surplus is promptly and easily eliminated. Trying to prevent the body from retaining water by drinking less is therefore not only futile but even harmful.

Constipation

An excess of water keeps the feces soft, and that is very important in the obese, who commonly suffer from constipation and a spastic colon. While a patient is under treatment we never permit the use of any kind of laxative taken by mouth. We explain that owing to the restricted diet it is perfectly satisfactory and normal to have an evacuation of the bowel only once every three to four days and that, provided plenty of fluids are taken, this never leads to any disturbance. Only in those patients who begin to fret after four days do we allow the use of a suppository. Patients who observe this rule find that after treatment they have a perfectly normal bowel action and this delights many of them almost as much as their loss of weight.

Investigating Dietary Errors

When the reason for a slight gain in weight is not immediately evident, it is necessary to investigate further. A patient who is unaware of having committed an error or is unwilling to admit a mistake protests indignantly when told he has done something he ought not to have done. In that atmosphere no fruitful investigation can be conducted; so we calmly explain that we are not accusing him of anything but that we know for certain from our not inconsiderable experience that something has gone wrong and that we must now sit down quietly together and try and find out what it was. Once the patient realizes that it is in his own interest that he play an active and not merely a passive role in this search, the reason for the setback is almost invariably discovered. Having been through hundreds of such sessions, we are nearly always able to distinguish the deliberate liar from the patient who is merely fooling himself or is really unaware of having erred.

Liars and Fools

When we see obese patients there are generally two of us present in order to speed up routine handling. Thus when we have to investigate a rise in weight, a glance is sufficient to make sure that we agree or disagree. If after a few questions we both feel reasonably sure that the patient is deliberately lying, we tell him that this is our opinion and warn him that unless he comes clean we may refuse further treatment. The way he reacts to this furnishes additional proof whether we are on the right track or not; we now very rarely make a mistake.

If the patient breaks down and confesses, we melt and are all forgiveness and treatment proceeds. Yet if such performances have to be repeated more than two or three times, we refuse further treatment. This happens in less than 1% of our cases. If the patient is stubborn and will not admit what he has been up to, we usually give him one more chance and continue even though we have been unable to find the reason for his gain. In many such cases there is no repetition, and frequently the patient does then confess a few days later after he has thought things over.

The patient who is fooling himself is the one who has committed some trifling, offense against the rules but who has been able to convince him that this is of no importance and cannot possibly account for the gain in weight. Women seem particularly prone to getting themselves entangled in such delusions. On the other hand, it does frequently happen that a patient will in the midst of a conversation unthinkingly spear an olive or forget that he has already eaten his breadstick.

A mother preparing food for the family may out of sheer habit forget that she must not taste the sauce to see whether it needs more salt. Sometimes a rich maiden aunt cannot be offended by refusing a cup of tea into which she has put two teaspoons of sugar, thoughtfully remembering the patient's taste from previous occasions. Such incidents are legion and are usually confessed without hesitation, but some patients seem genuinely able to forget these lapses and remember them with a visible shock only after insistent questioning.

In these cases we go carefully over the day. Sometimes the patient has been invited to a meal or gone to a restaurant, naively believing that the food has actually been prepared exactly according to instructions. They will say: "Yes, now that I come to think of it the steak did seem a bit bigger than the one I have at home, and it did taste better; maybe there was a little fat on it, though I specially told them to cut it all away". Sometimes the breadsticks were broken and a few fragments eaten, and "Maybe they were a little more than one". It is not uncommon for patients to place too much reliance on their memory of the diet-sheet and start eating carrots, beans or peas and then to seem genuinely surprised when their attention is called to the fact that these are forbidden, as they have not been listed.

Cosmetics

When no dietary error is elicited we turn to cosmetics. Most women find it hard to believe that fats, oils, creams and ointments applied to the skin are absorbed and interfere with weight reduction by HCG just as if they had been eaten. This almost incredible sensitivity to even such very minor increases in nutritional intake is a peculiar feature of the HCG method. For instance, we find that persons who habitually handle organic fats, such as workers in beauty parlors, masseurs, butchers, etc. never show what we consider a satisfactory loss of weight unless they can avoid fat coming into contact with their skin.

The point is so important that I will illustrate it with two cases. A lady who was cooperating perfectly suddenly increased half a pound. Careful questioning brought nothing to light. She had certainly made no dietary error nor had she used any kind of face cream, and she was already in the menopause. As we felt that we could trust her implicitly, we left the question suspended. Yet just as she was about to leave the consulting room she suddenly stopped, turned and snapped her fingers. "I've got it," she said. This is what had happened : She had bought herself a new set of make-up pots and bottles and, using her fingers, had transferred her large assortment of cosmetics to the new containers in anticipation of the day she would be able to use them again after her treatment.

The other case concerns a man who impressed us as being very conscientious. He was about 20 lbs. overweight but did not lose satisfactorily from the onset of treatment. Again and again we tried to find the reason but with no success, until one day he said:" I never told you this, but I have a glass eye. In fact, I have a whole set of them. I frequently change them, and every time I do that I put a special ointment in my eye socket. Do you think that could have anything to do with it?" As we thought just that, we asked him to stop using this ointment, and from that day on his weight-loss was regular.

We are particularly averse to those modern cosmetics which contain hormones, as any interference with endocrine regulations during treatment must be absolutely avoided. Many women whose skin has in the course of years become adjusted to the use of fat containing cosmetics find that their skin gets dry as soon as they stop using them. In such cases we permit the use of plain mineral oil, which has no nutritional value. On the other hand, mineral oil should not be used in preparing the food, first because of its undesirable laxative quality, and second because it absorbs some fat-soluble vitamins, which are then lost in the stool. We do permit the use of lipstick, powder and such lotions as are entirely free of fatty substances. We also allow brilliantine to be used on the hair but it must not be rubbed into the scalp. Obviously sun-tan oil is prohibited.

Many women are horrified when told that for the duration of treatment they cannot use face creams or have facial massages. They fear that this and the loss of weight will ruin their complexion. They can be fully reassured. Under treatment normal fat is restored to the skin, which rapidly becomes fresh and turgid, making the expression much more youthful. This is a characteristic of the HCG method which is a constant source of wonder to patients who have experienced or seen in others the facial ravages produced by the usual methods of reducing. An obese woman of 70 obviously cannot expect to have her pued face reduced to normal without a wrinkle, but it is remarkable how youthful her face remains in spite of her age.

The Voice

Incidentally, another interesting feature of the HCG method is that it does not ruin a singing voice. The typically obese prima donna usually finds that when she tries to reduce, the timbre of her voice is liable to change, and understandably this terrifies her. Under HCG this does not happen; indeed, in many cases the voice improves and the breathing invariably does. We have had many cases of professional singers very carefully controlled by expert voice teachers, and they have been so enthusiastic that they now frequently send us patients.

Other Reasons for a Gain

Apart from diet and cosmetics there can be a few other reasons for a small rise in weight. Some patients unwittingly take chewing gum, throat pastilles, vitamin pills, cough syrups etc., without realizing that the sugar or fats they contain may interfere with a regular loss of weight. Sex hormones or cortisone in its various modern forms must be avoided, though oral contraceptives are permitted. In fact the only self-medication we allow is aspirin for a headache, though headaches almost invariably disappear after a week of treatment, particularly if of the migraine type.

Occasionally we allow a sleeping tablet or a tranquilizer, but patients should be told that while under treatment they need and may get less sleep. For instance, here in Italy where it is customary to sleep during the siesta which lasts from one to four in the afternoon most patients find that though they lie down they are unable to sleep.

We encourage swimming and sun bathing during treatment, but it should be remembered that a severe sunburn always produces a temporary rise in weight, evidently due to water retention. The same may be seen when a patient gets a common cold during treatment. Finally, the weight can temporarily increase - paradoxical though this may sound - after an exceptional physical exertion of long duration leading to a feeling of exhaustion. A game of tennis, a vigorous swim, a run, a ride on horseback or a round of golf do not have this effect; but a long trek, a day of skiing, rowing or cycling or dancing into the small hours usually result in a gain of weight on the following day, unless the patient is in perfect training. In patients coming from abroad, where they always use their cars, we often see this effect after a strenuous day of shopping on foot, sightseeing and visits to galleries and museums. Though the extra muscular effort involved does consume some additional calories, this appears to be offset by the retention of water which the tired circulation cannot at once eliminate.

Appetite-reducing Drugs
We hardly ever use amphetamines, the appetite-reducing drugs such as Dexedrin, Dexamil, Preludin, etc., as there seems to be no need for them during the HCG treatment. The only time we find them useful is when a patient is, for impelling and unforeseen reasons, obliged to forego the injections for three to four days and yet wishes to continue the diet so that he need not interrupt the course.

Unforeseen Interruptions of Treatment
If an interruption of treatment lasting more than four days is necessary, the patient must increase his diet to at least 800 calories by adding meat, eggs, cheese, and milk to his diet after the third day, as otherwise he will find himself so hungry and weak that he is unable to go about his usual occupation. If the interval lasts less than two weeks the patient can directly resume injections and the 500-calorie diet, but if the interruption lasts longer he must again eat normally until he has had his third injection.

When a patient knows beforehand that he will have to travel and be absent for more than four days, it is always better to stop injections three days before he is due to leave so that he can have the three days of strict dieting which are necessary after the last injection at home. This saves him from the almost impossible task of having to arrange the 500 calorie diet while en route, and he can thus enjoy a much greater dietary freedom from the day of his departure. Interruptions occurring before 20 effective injections have been given are most undesirable, because with less than that number of injections some weight is liable to be regained. After the 20th injection an unavoidable interruption is merely a loss of time.

Muscular Fatigue
Towards the end of a full course, when a good deal of fat has been rapidly lost, some patients complain that lifting a weight or climbing stairs requires a greater muscular effort than before. They feel neither breathlessness nor exhaustion but simply that their muscles have to work harder. This phenomenon, which disappears soon after the end of the treatment, is caused by the removal of abnormal fat deposited between, in, and around the muscles. The removal of this fat makes the muscles too long, and so in order to achieve a certain skeletal movement - say the bending of an arm - the muscles have to perform greater contraction than before. Within a short while the muscle adjusts itself perfectly to the new situation, but under HCG the loss of fat is so rapid that this adjustment cannot keep up with it. Patients often have to be reassured that this does not mean that they are "getting weak". This phenomenon does not occur in patients who regularly take vigorous exercise and continue to do so during treatment.

Massage
I never allow any kind of massage during treatment. It is entirely unnecessary and merely disturbs a very delicate process which is going on in the tissues. Few indeed are the masseurs and masseuses who can resist the temptation to knead and hammer abnormal fat deposits. In the course of rapid reduction it is sometimes possible to pick up a fold of skin which has not yet had time to adjust itself, as it always does under HCG, to the changed figure. This fold contains its normal subcutaneous fat and may be almost an inch thick. It is one of the main objects of the HCG treatment to keep that fat there. Patients and their masseurs do not always understand this and give this fat a working-over. I have seen such patients who were as black and blue as if they had received a sound thrashing.

In my opinion, massage, thumping, rolling, kneading, and shivering undertaken for the purpose of reducing abnormal fat can do nothing but harm. We once had the honor of treating the proprietress of a high class institution that specialized in such antics. She had the audacity to confess that she was taking our treatment to convince her clients of the efficacy of her methods, which she had found useless in her own case.

How anyone in his right mind is able to believe that fatty tissue can be shifted mechanically or be made to vanish by squeezing is beyond my comprehension. The only effect obtained is severe bruising. The torn tissue then forms scars and these slowly contracts making the fatty tissue even harder and more unyielding.

A lady once consulted us for her most ungainly legs. Large masses of fat bulged over the ankles of her tiny feet, and there were about 40 lbs. too much on her hips and thighs. We assured her that this overweight could be lost and that her ankles would markedly improve in the process. Her treatment progressed most satisfactorily but to our surprise there was no improvement in her ankles. We then discovered that she had for years been taking every kind of mechanical, electric and heat treatment for her legs and that she had made up her mind to resort to plastic surgery if we failed.

Re-examining the fat above her ankles, we found that it was unusually hard. We attributed this to the countless minor injuries inflicted by kneading. These injuries had healed but had left a tough network of connective scar-tissue in which the fat was imprisoned. Ready to try anything, she was put to bed for the remaining three weeks of her first course with her lower legs tightly strapped in unyielding bandages. Every day the pressure was increased. The combination of HCG, diet and strapping brought about a marked improvement in the shape of her ankles. At the end of her first course she returned to her home abroad. Three months later she came back for her second course. She had maintained both her weight and the improvement of her ankles. The same procedure was repeated, and after five weeks she left the hospital with a normal weight and legs that, if not exactly shapely, were at least unobtrusive. Where no such injuries of the tissues have been inflicted by inappropriate methods of treatment, these drastic measures are never necessary.

Blood Sugar
Towards the end of a course or when a patient has nearly reached his normal weight it occasionally happens that the blood sugar drops below normal, and we have even seen this in patients who had an abnormally high blood sugar before treatment. Such an attack of hypoglycemia is almost identical with the one seen in diabetics who have taken too much insulin. The attack comes on suddenly; there is the same feeling of light-headedness, weakness in the knees, trembling, and unmotivated sweating. But under HCG, hypoglycemia does not produce any feeling of hunger. All these symptoms are almost instantly relieved by taking two heaped teaspoons of sugar.

In the course of treatment the possibility of such an attack is explained to those patients who are in a phase in which a drop in blood sugar may occur. They are instructed to keep sugar or glucose sweets handy, particularly when driving a car. They are also told to watch the effect of taking sugar very carefully and report the following day. This is important, because anxious patients to whom such an attack has been explained are apt to take sugar unnecessarily, in which case it inevitably produces a gain in weight and does not dramatically relieve the symptoms for which it was taken, proving that these were not due to hypoglycemia. Some patients mistake the effects of emotional stress for hypoglycemia. When the symptoms are quickly relieved by sugar this is proof that they were indeed due to an abnormal lowering of the blood sugar, and in that case there is no increase in the weight on the following day. We always suggest that sugar be taken if the patient is in doubt.

Once such an attack has been relieved with sugar we have never seen it recur on the immediately subsequent days, and only very rarely does a patient have two such attacks separated by several days during a course of treatment. In patients who have not eaten sufficiently during the first two days of treatment we sometimes give sugar when the minor symptoms usually felt during the first there days of treatment continue beyond that time, and in some cases this has seemed to speed up the euphoria ordinarily associated with the HCG method.

The Ratio of Pounds to Inches
An interesting feature of the HCG method is that, regardless of how fat a patient is, the greatest circumference -- abdomen or hips as the case may be is reduced at a constant rate which is extraordinarily close to 1 cm. per kilogram of weight lost. At the beginning of treatment the change in measurements is somewhat greater than this, but at the end

of a course it is almost invariably found that the girth is as many centimeters less as the number of kilograms by which the weight has been reduced. I have never seen this clear cut relationship in patients that try to reduce by dieting only.

Preparing the Solution

Human chorionic gonadotrophin comes on the market as a highly soluble powder which is the pure substance extracted from the urine of pregnant women. Such preparations are carefully standardized, and any brand made by a reliable pharmaceutical company is probably as good as any other. The substance should be extracted from the urine and not from the placenta, and it must of course be of human and not of animal origin. The powder is sealed in ampoules or in rubber-capped bottles in varying amounts which are stated in International Units. In this form HCG is stable; however, only such preparations should be used that have the date of manufacture and the date of expiry clearly stated on the label or package. A suitable solvent is always supplied in a separate ampoule in the same package.

Once HCG is in solution it is far less stable. It may be kept at room-temperature for two to three days, but if the solution must be kept longer it should always be refrigerated. When treating only one or two cases simultaneously, vials containing a small number of units say 1000 I.U. should be used. The 10 cc. of solvent which is supplied by the manufacturer is injected into the rubber- capped bottle containing the HCG, and the powder must dissolve instantly. Of this solution 1 .25 cc. are withdrawn for each injection. One such bottle of 1000 I.U. therefore furnishes 8 injections. When more than one patient is being treated, they should not each have their own bottle but rather all be injected from the same vial and a fresh solution made when this is empty.

As we are usually treating a fair number of patients at the same time, we prefer to use vials containing 5000 units. With these the manufactures also supply 10 cc. of solvent. Of such a solution 0.25 cc. contain the 125 I.U., which is the standard dose for all cases and which should never be exceeded. This small amount is awkward to handle accurately (it requires an insulin syringe) and is wasteful, because there is a loss of solution in the nozzle of the syringe and in the needle. We therefore prefer a higher dilution, which we prepare in the following way: The solvent supplied is injected into the rubber-capped bottle containing the 5000 I.U . As these bottles are too small to hold more solvent, we withdraw 5 cc., inject it into an empty rubber-capped bottle and add 5 cc. of normal saline to each bottle. This gives us 10 cc. of solution in each bottle, and of this solution 0.5 cc. contains 125 I.U. This amount is convenient to inject with an ordinary syringe.

Injecting

HCG produces little or no tissue-reaction, it is completely painless and in the many thousands of injections we have given we have never seen an inflammatory or suppurative reaction at the site of the injection.

One should avoid leaving a vacuum in the bottle after preparing the solution or after withdrawal of the amount required for the injections as otherwise alcohol used for sterilizing a frequently perforated rubber cap might be drawn into the solution. When sharp needles are used, it sometimes happens that a little bit of rubber is punched out of the rubber cap and can be seen as a small black speck floating in the solution. As these bits of rubber are heavier than the solution they rapidly settle out, and it is thus easy to avoid drawing them into the syringe.

We use very fine needles that are two inches long and inject deep intragluteally in the outer upper quadrant of the buttocks. The injection should if possible not be given into the superficial fat layers, which in very obese patients must be compressed so as to enable the needle to reach the muscle. It is also important that the daily injection should be given at intervals as close to 24 hours as possible. Any attempt to economize in time by giving larger doses at longer intervals is doomed to produce less satisfactory results.

There are hardly any contraindications to the HCG method. Treatment can be continued in the presence of abscesses, suppuration, large infected wounds and major fractures. Surgery and general anesthesia are no reason to stop and we have given treatment during a severe attack of malaria. Acne or boils are no contraindication, the former usually clears up, and furunculosis comes to an end. Thrombophlebitis is no contraindication, and we have treated several obese patients with HCG and the 500-calorie diet while suffering from this condition. Our impression has been that in obese patients the phlebitis does rather better and certainly no worse than under the usual treatment alone. This also applies to patients suffering from varicose ulcers which tend to heal rapidly.

Fibroids

While uterine fibroids seem to be in no way affected by HCG in the doses we use, we have found that very large, externally palpable uterine myomas are apt to give trouble. We are convinced that this is entirely due to the rather sudden disappearance of fat from the pelvic bed upon which they rest and that it is the weight of the tumor pressing on the underlying tissues which accounts for the discomfort or pain which may arise during treatment. While we disregard even fair-sized or multiple myomas, we insist that very large ones be operated before treatment. We have had patients present themselves for reducing fat from their abdomen who showed no signs of obesity, but had a large abdominal tumor.

Gallstones

Small stones in the gall bladder may in patients who have recently had typical colics cause more frequent colics under treatment with HCG. This may be due to the almost complete absence of fat from the diet, which prevents the normal emptying of the gall bladder. Before undertaking treatment we explain to such patients that there is a risk of more frequent and possibly severe symptoms and that it may become necessary to operate. If they are prepared to take this risk and provided they agree to undergo an operation if we consider this imperative, we proceed with treatment, as after weight reduction with HCG the operative risk is considerably reduced in an obese patient. In such cases we always give a drug which stimulates the flow of bile, and in the majority of cases nothing untoward happens. On the other hand, we have looked for and not found any evidence to suggest that the HCG treatment leads to the formation of gallstones as pregnancy sometimes does.

The Heart

Disorders of the heart are not as a rule contraindications. In fact, the removal of abnormal fat - particularly from the heart-muscle and from the surrounding of the coronary arteries - can only be beneficial in cases of myocardial weakness, and many such patients are referred to us by cardiologists. Within the first week of treatment all patients - not only heart cases - remark that they have lost much of their breathlessness

Coronary Occlusion

In obese patients who have recently survived a coronary occlusion, we adopt the following procedure in collaboration with the cardiologist. We wait until no further electrocardiographic changes have occurred for a period of three months. Routine treatment is then started under careful control and it is usual to find a further electrocardiographic improvement of a condition which was previously stationary.

In the thousands of cases we have treated we have not once seen any sort of coronary incident occur during or shortly after treatment. The same applies to cerebral vascular accidents. Nor have we ever seen a case of thrombosis of any sort develop during treatment, even though a high blood pressure is rapidly lowered. In this respect, too, the HCG treatment resembles pregnancy.

Teeth and Vitamins

Patients whose teeth are in poor repair sometimes get more trouble under prolonged treatment, just as may occur in pregnancy. In such cases we do allow calcium and vitamin D, though not in an oily solution. The only other vitamin we permit is vitamin C, which we use in large doses combined with an antihistamine at the onset of a common cold. There is no objection to the use of an antibiotic if this is required, for instance by the dentist. In cases of bronchial asthma and hay fever we have occasionally resorted to cortisone during treatment and find that triamcinolone is the least likely to interfere with the loss of weight, but many asthmatics improve with HCG alone.

Alcohol

Obese heavy drinkers, even those bordering on alcoholism, often do surprisingly well under HCG and it is exceptional for them to take a drink while under treatment. When they do, they find that a relatively small quantity of alcohol produces intoxication. Such patients say that they do not feel the need to drink This may in part be due to the euphoria which the treatment produces and in part to the complete absence of the need for quick sustenance from which most obese patients suffer.

Though we have had a few cases that have continued abstinence long after treatment, others relapse as soon as they are back on a normal diet. We have a few "regular customers" who, having once been reduced to their normal weight, start to drink again though watching their weight. Then after some months they purposely overeat in order to gain sufficient weight for another course of HCG which temporarily gets them out of their drinking routine. We do not particularly welcome such cases, but we see no reason for refusing their request.

Tuberculosis

It is interesting that obese patients suffering from inactive pulmonary tuberculosis can be safely treated. We have under very careful control treated patients as early as three months after they were pronounced inactive and have never seen a relapse occur during or shortly after treatment. In fact, we only have one case on our records in which active tuberculosis developed in a young man about one year after a treatment which had lasted three weeks. Earlier X-rays showed a calcified spot from a childhood infection which had not produced clinical symptoms. There was a family history of tuberculosis, and his illness started under adverse conditions which certainly had nothing to do with the treatment. Residual calcifications from an early infection are exceedingly common, and we never consider them a contraindication to treatment.

The Painful Heel

In obese patients who have been trying desperately to keep their weight down by severe dieting, a curious symptom sometimes occurs. They complain of an unbearable pain in their heels which they feel only while standing or walking. As soon as they take the weight off their heels the pain ceases. These cases are the bane of the rheumatologists and orthopedic surgeons who have treated them before they come to us. All the usual investigations are entirely negative, and there is not the slightest response to anti- rheumatic medication or physiotherapy. The pain may be so severe that the patients are obliged to give up their occupation, and they are not infrequently labeled as a case of hysteria. When their heels are carefully examined one finds that the sole is softer than normal and that the heel bone - the calcaneus - can be distinctly felt, which is not the case in a normal foot.

We interpret the condition as a lack of the hard fatty pad on which the calcaneus rests and which protects both the bone and the skin of the sole from pressure. This fat is like a springy cushion which carries the weight of the body. Standing on a heel in which this fat is missing or reduced must obviously be very painful. In their efforts to keep their weight down these patients have consumed this normal structural fat.

Those patients who have a normal or subnormal weight while showing the typically obese fat deposits are made to eat to capacity, often much against their will, for one week. They gain weight rapidly but there is no improvement in the painful heels. They are then started on the routine HCG treatment. Overweight patients are treated immediately. In both cases the pain completely disappears in 10-20 days of dieting, usually around the 15th day of treatment, and so far no case has had a relapse. We have been able to follow up such patients for years.

We are particularly interested in these cases, as they furnish further proof of the contention that HCG + 500 calories not only removes abnormal fat but actually permits normal fat to be replaced, in spite of the deficient food intake. It is certainly not so that the mere loss of weight reduces the pain, because it frequently disappears before the weight the patient had prior to the period of forced feeding is reached.

The Skeptical Patient

Any doctor who starts using the HCG method for the first time will have considerable difficulty, particularly if he himself is not fully convinced, in making patients believe that they will not feel hungry on 500 calories and that their face will not collapse. New patients always anticipate the phenomena they know so well from previous treatments and diets and are incredulous when told that these will not occur. We overcome all this by letting new patients spend a little time in the waiting room with older hands, who can always be relied upon to allay these fears with evangelistic zeal, often demonstrating the finer points on their own body.

A waiting-room filled with obese patients who congregate daily is a sort of group therapy. They compare notes and pop back into the waiting room after the consultation to announce the score of the last 24 hours to an enthralled audience. They cross-check on their diets and sometimes confess sins which they try to hide from us, usually with the result that the patient in whom they have confided palpitatingly tattles the whole disgraceful story to us with a "But don't let her know I told you."

Concluding a Course

When the three days of dieting after the last injection are over, the patients are told that they may now eat anything they please, except sugar and starch provided they faithfully observe one simple rule. This rule is that they must have their own portable bathroom-scale always at hand, particularly while traveling. They must without fail weight themselves every morning as they get out of bed, having first emptied their bladder. If they are in the habit of having breakfast in bed, they must weigh before breakfast.

It takes about 3 weeks before the weight reached at the end of the treatment becomes stable, i.e. does not show violent fluctuations after an occasional excess. During this period patients must realize that the so-called carbohydrates, that is sugar, rice, bread, potatoes, pastries etc, are by far the most dangerous. If no carbohydrates whatsoever are eaten, fats can be indulged in somewhat more liberally and even small quantities of alcohol, such as a glass of wine with meals, does no harm, but **as soon as fats and starch are combined things are very liable to get out of hand.** This has to be observed very carefully during the first 3 weeks after the treatment is ended otherwise disappointments are almost sure to occur.

Skipping a Meal

As long as their weight stays within two pounds of the weight reached on the day of the last injection, patients should take no notice of any increase but the moment the scale goes beyond two pounds, even if this is only a few ounces, they must on that same day entirely skip breakfast and lunch but take plenty to drink. In the evening they must eat a huge steak with only an apple or a raw tomato. Of course this rule applies only to the morning weight. Ex-obese patients should never check their weight during the day, as there may be wide fluctuations and these are merely alarming and confusing.

It is of utmost importance that the meal is skipped on the same day as the scale registers an increase of more than two pounds and that missing the meals is not postponed until the following day. If a meal is skipped on the day in which a gain is registered in the morning this brings about an immediate drop of often over a pound. But if the skipping of the meal - and skipping means literally skipping, not just having a light meal - is postponed the phenomenon does not occur and several days of strict dieting may be necessary to correct the situation.

Most patients hardly ever need to skip a meal. If they have eaten a heavy lunch they feel no desire to eat their dinner, and in this case no increase takes place. If they keep their weight at the point reached at the end of the treatment, even a heavy dinner does not bring about an increase of two pounds on the next morning and does not therefore call for any special measures. Most patients are surprised how small their appetite has become and yet how much they can eat without gaining weight. They no longer suffer from an abnormal appetite and feel satisfied with much less food than before. In fact, they are usually disappointed that they cannot manage their first normal meal, which they have been planning for weeks.

Losing more Weight

An ex-patient should never gain more than two pounds without immediately correcting this, but it is equally undesirable that more than two pounds be lost after treatment, because a greater loss is always achieved at the expense of normal fat. Any normal fat that is lost is invariably regained as soon as more food is taken, and it often happens that this rebound overshoots the upper two lbs. limit.

- 34 -

Trouble After Treatment

Two difficulties may be encountered in the immediate post-treatment period. When a patient has consumed all his abnormal fat or, when after a full course, the injection has temporarily lost its efficacy owing to the body having gradually evolved a counter regulation, the patient at once begins to feel much more hungry and even weak. In spite of repeated warnings, some over-enthusiastic patients do not report this. However, in about two days the fact that they are being undernourished becomes visible in their faces, and treatment is then stopped at once. In such cases - and only in such cases - we allow a very slight increase in the diet, such as an extra apple, 150 grams of meat or two or three extra breadsticks during the three days of dieting after the last injection.

When abnormal fat is no longer being put into circulation either because it has been consumed or because immunity has set in, this is always felt by the patient as sudden, intolerable and constant hunger. In this sense, the HCG method is completely self-limiting. With HCG it is impossible to reduce a patient, however enthusiastic, beyond his normal weight. As soon as no more abnormal fat is being issued, the body starts consuming normal fat, and this is always regained as soon as ordinary feeding is resumed. The patient then finds that the 2-3 lbs. he has lost during the last days of treatment are immediately regained. A meal is skipped and maybe a pound is lost. The next day this pound is regained, in spite of a careful watch over the food intake. In a few days a tearful patient is back in the consulting room, convinced that her case is a failure.

All that is happening is that the essential fat lost at the end of the treatment, owing to the patient's reluctance to report a much greater hunger, is being replaced. The weight at which such a patient must stabilize thus lies 2-3 lbs. higher than the weight reached at the end of the treatment. Once this higher basic level is established, further difficulties in controlling the weight at the new point of stabilization hardly arise.

Beware of Over-enthusiasm

The other trouble which is frequently encountered immediately after treatment is again due to over-enthusiasm. Some patients cannot believe that they can eat fairly normally without regaining weight. They disregard the advice to eat anything they please except sugar and starch and want to play safe. They try more or less to continue the 500-calorie diet on which they felt so well during treatment and make only minor variations, such as replacing the meat with an egg, cheese, or a glass of milk. To their horror they find that in spite of this bravura, their weight goes up. So, following instructions, they skip one meager lunch and at night eat only a little salad and drink a pot of unsweetened tea, becoming increasingly hungry and weak. The next morning they find that they have increased yet another pound. They feel terrible, and even the dreaded swelling of their ankles is back. Normally we check our patients one week after they have been eating freely, but these cases return in a few days. Either their eyes are filled with tears or they angrily imply that when we told them to eat normally we were just fooling them.

Protein deficiency

Here too, the explanation is quite simple. During treatment the patient has been only just above the verge of protein deficiency and has had the advantage of protein being fed back into his system from the breakdown of fatty tissue. Once the treatment is over there is no more HCG in the body and this process no longer takes place. Unless an adequate amount of protein is eaten as soon as the treatment is over, protein deficiency is bound to develop, and this inevitably causes the marked retention of water known as hunger- edema.

The treatment is very simple. The patient is told to eat two eggs for breakfast and a huge steak for lunch and dinner followed by a large helping of cheese and to phone through the weight the next morning. When these instructions are followed a stunned voice is heard to report that two lbs. have vanished overnight, that the ankles are normal but that sleep was disturbed, owing to an extraordinary need to pass large quantities of water. The patient having learned this lesson usually has no further trouble.

Relapses

As a general rule one can say that 60%-70% of our cases experience little or no difficulty in holding their weight permanently. Relapses may be due to negligence in the basic rule of daily weighing. Many patients think that this is unnecessary and that they can judge any increase from the fit of their clothes. Some do not carry their scale with them on a journey as it is cumbersome and takes a big bite out of their luggage-allowance when flying. This is a disastrous mistake, because after a course of HCG as much as 10 lbs. can be regained without any noticeable change in the fit of the clothes. The reason for this is that after treatment newly acquired fat is at first evenly distributed and does not show the former preference for certain parts of the body.

Pregnancy or the menopause may annul the effect of a previous treatment. Women who take treatment during the one year after the last menstruation - that is at the onset of the menopause - do just as well as others, but among them the relapse rate is higher until the menopause is fully established. The period of one year after the last menstruation applies only to women who are not being treated with ovarian hormones. If these are taken, the premenopausal period may be indefinitely prolonged.

Late teenage girls who suffer from attacks of compulsive eating have by far the worst record of all as far as relapses are concerned.

Patients who have once taken the treatment never seem to hesitate to come back for another short course as soon as they notice that their weight is once again getting out of hand. They come quite cheerfully and hopefully, assured that they can be helped again. Repeat courses are often even more satisfactory than the first treatment and have the advantage, as do second courses, that the patient already, knows that he will feel comfortable throughout.

Plan of a Normal Course

125 I.U. of HCG daily (except during menstruation) iu injections have been given.

Until 3rd injection forced feeding.

After 3rd injection, 500 calorie diet to be continued until 72 hours after the last injection.

For the following 3 weeks, all foods allowed except starch and sugar in any form (careful with very sweet fruit).

After 3 weeks, very gradually add starch in small quantities, always controlled by morning weighing.

CONCLUSION

The HCG + diet method can bring relief to every case of obesity, but the method is not simple. It is very time consuming and requires perfect cooperation between physician and patient. Each case must be handled individually, and the physician must have time to answer questions, allay fears and remove misunderstandings. He must also check the patient daily. When something goes wrong he must at once investigate until he finds the reason for any gain that may have occurred. In most cases it is useless to hand the patient a diet-sheet and let the nurse give him a "shot."

The method involves a highly complex bodily mechanism, and the physician must make himself some sort of picture of what is actually happening; otherwise he will not be able to deal with such difficulties as may arise during treatment.

I must beg those trying the method for the first time to adhere very strictly to the technique and the interpretations here outlined and thus treat a few hundred cases before embarking on experiments of their own, and until then refrain from introducing innovations, however thrilling they may seem. In a new method, innovations or departures from the original technique can only be usefully evaluated against a substantial background of experience with what is at the moment the orthodox procedure.

I have tried to cover all the problems that come to my mind. Yet a bewildering array of new questions keeps arising, and my interpretations are still fluid. In particular, I have never had an opportunity of conducting the laboratory investigations which are so necessary for a theoretical understanding of clinical observations, and I can only hope that those more fortunately placed will in time be able to fill this gap.

The problems of obesity are perhaps not so dramatic as the problems of cancer, but they often cause life long suffering. How many promising careers have been ruined by excessive fat; how many lives have been shortened. If some way -however cumbersome - can be found to cope effectively with this universal problem of modern civilized man, our world will be a happier place for countless fellow men and women.

GLOSSARY

ACNE . . . Common skin disease in which pimples, often containing pus, appear on face, neck and shoulders.

ACTH . . . Abbreviation for adrenocorticotrophic hormone. One of the many hormones produced by the anterior lobe of the pituitary gland. ACTH controls the outer part, rind or cortex of the adrenal glands. When ACTH is injected it dramatically relieves arthritic pain, but it has many undesirable side effects, among which is a condition similar to severe obesity. ACTH is now usually replaced by cortisone.

ADRENALIN . . . Hormone produced by the inner part of the Adrenals. Among many other functions, adrenalin is concerned with blood pressure, emotional stress, fear and cold.

ADRENALS . . . Endocrine glands. Small bodies situated atop the kidneys and hence also known as suprarenal glands. The adrenals have an outer rind or cortex which produces vitally important hormones, among which are Cortisone similar substances. The adrenal cortex is controlled by ACTH. The inner part of the adrenals, the medulla, secretes adrenalin and is chiefly controlled by the autonomous nervous system.

ADRENOCORTEX... See adrenals.

AMPHETAMINES . . . Synthetic drugs which reduce the awareness of hunger and stimulate mental activity, rendering sleep impossible. When used for the latter two purposes they are dangerously habit-forming. They do not diminish the body's need for food, but merely suppress the perception of that need. The original drug was known as Benzedrine, from which modern variants such as Dexedrine, Dexamil, and Preludin have been derived. Amphetamines may help an obese patient to prevent a further increase in weight but are unsatisfactory for reducing, as they do not cure the underlying disorder and as their prolonged use may lead to malnutrition and addiction.

ARTERIOSCLEROSIS . . . Hardening of the arterial wall through the calcification of abnormal deposits of a fatlike substance known as cholesterol.

ASCHFIE1M-ZONDEK . . . Authors of a test by which early pregnancy can be diagnosed by injecting a woman's urine into female mice. The HCG present in pregnancy urine produces certain changes in the vagina of these animals. Many similar tests, using other animals such as rabbits, frogs, etc. have been devised.

ASSIMILATE . . . Absorbed digested food from the intestines.

AUTONOMOUS . . . Here used to describe the independent or vegetative nervous system which manages the automatic regulations of the body.

BASAL METABOLISM . . . The body's chemical turnover at complete rest and when fasting. The basal metabolic rate is expressed as the amount of oxygen used up in a given time. The basal metabolic rate (BMR) is controlled by the thyroid gland.

CALORIE . . . The physicist's calorie is the amount of heat required to raise the temperature of 1 cc. of water by 1 degree Centigrade. The dieticiari's Calorie (always written with a capital C) is 1000 times greater. Thus when we speak of a 500 Calorie diet this means that the body is being supplied with as much fuel as would be required to raise the temperature of 500 liters of water by 1 degree Centigrade or 50 liters by 10 degrees. This is quite insufficient to cover the heat and energy requirements of an adult body. In the HCG method the deficit is made up from the abnormal fat-deposits, of which 1 lb. furnishes the body with more than 2000 Calories. As this is roughly the amount lost every day, a patient under HCG is never short of fuel.

CEREBRAL . . . Of the brain. Cerebral vascular disease is a disorder concerning the blood vessels of the brain, such as cerebral thrombosis or hemorrhage, known as apoplexy or stroke.

CHOLESTEROL . . . A fatlike substance contained in almost every cell of the body. In the blood it exists in two forms, known as free and esterified. The latter form is under certain conditions deposited in the inner lining of the arteries (see arteriosclerosis). No clear and definite relationship between fat intake and cholesterol-level in the blood has yet been established.

CHORIONIC . . . Of the chorion, which is part of the placenta or after-birth. The term chorionic is justly applied to HCG, as this hormone is exclusively produced in the placenta, from where it enters the human mother's blood and is later excreted in her urine.

COMPULSIVE EATING. . . A form of oral gratification with which a repressed sex-instinct is sometimes vicariously relieved. Compulsive eating must not be confused with the real hunger from which most obese patients suffer.

CONGENITAL . . . Any condition which exists at or before birth.

CORONARY ARTERIES . . . Two blood vessels which encircle the heart and supply all the blood required by the heart-muscle.

CORPUS LUTEUM . . . A yellow body which forms in the ovary at the follicle from which an egg has been detached. This body acts as an endocrine gland and plays an important role in menstruation and pregnancy. Its secretion is one of the sex hormones, and it is stimulated by another hormone known as LSH, which stands for luteum stimulating hormones. LSH is produced in the anterior lobe of the pituitary gland. LSH is truly gonadotrophic and must never be confused with HCG, which is a totally different substance, having no direct action on the corpus luteum.

CORTEX . . . Outer covering or rind. The term is applied to the outer part of the adrenals but is also used to describe the gray matter which covers the white matter of the brain.

CORTISONE . . . A synthetic substance which acts like an adrenal hormone. It is today used in the treatment of a large number of illnesses, and several chemical variants have been produced, among which are prednisone and triaincinolone.

CUSHING . . . A great American brain surgeon who described a condition of extreme obesity associated with symptoms of adrenal disorder. Cushing's Syndrome may be caused by organic disease of the pituitary or the adrenal glands but, as was later discovered, it also occurs as a result of excessive ACTH medication.

DIENCEPHALON . . . A primitive and hence very old part of the brain which lies between and under the two large hemispheres. In man the diencephalon (or hypothalamus) is subordinate to the higher brain or cortex, and yet it ultimately controls all that happens inside the body. It regulates all the endocrine glands, the autonomous nervous system, the turnover of fat and sugar. It seems also to be the seat of the primitive animal instincts and is the relay station at which emotions are translated into bodily reactions.

DIURETIC. . . Any substance that increases the flow of urine.

DYSFUNCTION . . . Abnormal functioning of any organ, be this excessive, deficient or in any way altered.

EDEMA . . . An abnormal accumulation of water in the tissues.

ELECTROCARDIOGRAM . . . Tracing of electric phenomena taking place in the heart during each beat. The tracing provides information about the condition and working of the heart which is not otherwise obtainable.

ENDOCRINE . . . We distinguish endocrine and exocrine glands. The former produce hormones, chemical regulators, which they secrete directly into the blood circulation in the gland and from where they are carried all over the body. Examples of endocrine glands are the pituitary, the thyroid and the adrenals. Exocrine glands produce a visible secretion such as saliva, sweat, urine. There are also glands which are endocrine and exocrine. Examples are the testicles, the prostate and the pancreas, which produces the hormone insulin and digestive ferments which flow from the gland into the intestinal tract. Endocrine glands are closely inter dependent of each other, they are linked to the autonomous nervous system and the diencephalon presides over this whole incredibly complex regulatory system.

EMACIATED . . . Grossly undernourished.

EUPHORIA . . . A feeling of particular physical and mental well being.

FERAL . . . Wild, unrestrained.

FIBROID . . . Any benign new growth of connective tissue. When such a tumor originates from a muscle, it is known as a myoma. The most common seat of myomas is the uterus.

FOLLICLE . . . Any small bodily cyst or sac containing a liquid. Here the term applies to the ovarian cyst in which the egg is formed. The egg is expelled when a ripe follicle bursts and this is known as ovulation (see corpus luteurn).

FSH . . . Abbreviation for follicle-stimulating hormone. FSH is another (see corpus luteum) anterior pituitary hormone which acts directly on the ovarian follicle and is therefore correctly called a gonadotrophin.

GLANDS . . . See endocrine.

GONADOTROPHIN . . . See corpus luteum, follicle and FSH. Gonadotrophic literally means sex gland-directed. FSH, LSH and the equivalent hormones in the male, all produced in the anterior lobe of the pituitary gland, are true gonadotrophins. Unfortunately and confusingly, the term gonadotrophin has also been applied to the placental hormone of pregnancy known as human chorionic gonadotrophin (HCG). This hormone acts on the diencephalon and can only indirectly influence the sex-glands via the anterior lobe of the pituitary.

HCG . . . Abbreviation for human chorionic gonadotrophin

HORMONES . . . See endocrine.

HYPERTENSION . . . High blood pressure.

HYPOGLYCEMIA . . . A condition in which the blood sugar is below normal. It can be relieved by eating sugar.

HYPOPHYSIS . . . Another name for the pituitary gland.

HYPOTHESIS . . . A tentative explanation or speculation on how observed facts and isolated scientific data can be brought into an intellectually satisfying relationship of cause and effect. Hypotheses are useful for directing further research, but they are not necessarily an exposition of what is believed to be the truth. Before a hypothesis can advance to the dignity of a theory or a law, it must be confirmed by all future research. As soon as research turns up data which no longer fit the hypothesis, it is immediately abandoned for a better one.

LSH . . . See corpus luteum.

METABOLISM . . . See basal metabolism.

MIGRAINE . . . Severe half-sided headache often associated with vomiting.

MUCOID . . . Slime-like.

MYOCARDIUM . . . The heart-muscle.

MYOMA . . . See fibroid.

MYXEDEMA . . . Accumulation of a mucoid substance in the tissues which occurs in cases of severe primary thyroid deficiency.

NEOLITHIC . . . In the history of human culture we distinguish the Early Stone Age or Paleolithic, the Middle Stone Age or Mesolithic and the New Stone Age or Neolithic period. The Neolithic period started about 8000 years ago when the first attempts at agriculture, pottery and animal domestication made at the end of the Mesolithic period suddenly began to develop rapidly along the road that led to modern civilization.

NORMAL SALINE . . . A low concentration of salt in water equal to the salinity of body fluids.

PHLEBITIS . . . An inflammation of the veins. When a blood-clot forms at the site of the inflammation, we speak of thrombophlebitis.

PITUITARY . . . A very complex endocrine gland which lies at the base of the skull, consisting chiefly of an anterior and a posterior lobe. The pituitary is controlled by the diencephalon, which regulates the anterior lobe by means of hormones which reach it through small blood vessels. The posterior lobe is controlled by nerves which run from the diencephalon into this part of the gland. The anterior lobe secretes many hormones, among which are those that regulate other glands such as the thyroid, the adrenals and the sex glands.

PLACENTA . . . The after-birth. In women, a large and highly complex organ through which the child in the womb receives its nourishment from the mother's body. It is the organ in which HCG is manufactured and then given off into the mother's blood.

PROTEIN . . . The living substance in plant and animal cells. Herbivorous animals can thrive on plant protein alone, but man must base some protein of animal origin (milk, eggs or flesh) to live healthily. When insufficient protein is eaten, the body retains water.

PSORIASIS . . . A skin disease which produces scaly patches. These tend to disappear during pregnancy and during the treatment of obesity by the HCG method.

RENAL . . . Of the kidney.

RESERPINE . . . An Indian drug extensively used in the treatment of high blood pressure and some forms of mental disorder.

RETENTION ENEMA . . . The slow infusion of a liquid into the rectum, from where it is absorbed and not evacuated.

SACRUM . . . A fusion of the lower vertebrate into the large bony mass to which the pelvis is attached.

SEDIMENTATION RATE . . . The speed at which a suspension of red blood cells settles out. A rapid settling out is called a high sedimentation rate and may be indicative of a large number of bodily disorders of pregnancy.

SEXUAL SELECTION . . . A sexual preference for individuals which show certain traits. If this preference or selection goes on generation after generation, more and more individuals showing the trait will appear among the general population. The natural environment has little or nothing to do with this process. Sexual selection therefore differs from natural selection, to which modern man is no longer subject because he changes his environment rather than let the environment change him.

STRIATION . . . Tearing of the lower layers of the skin owing to rapid stretching in obesity or during pregnancy. When first formed striae are dark reddish lines which later change into white scars.

SUPRARENAL GLANDS . . . See adrenals.

SYNDROME . . . A group of symptoms which in their association are characteristic of a particular disorder.

THROMBOPHLEBITIS . . . See phlebitis.

THROMBUS . . . A blood-clot in a blood-vessel.

TRIAMCINOLONE . . . A modern derivative of cortisone.

URIC ACID . . . A product of incomplete protein-breakdown or utilization in the body. When uric acid becomes deposited in the gristle of the joints we speak of gout.

VARICOSE ULCERS . . . Chronic ulceration above the ankles due to varicose veins which interfere with the normal blood circulation in the affected areas.

VEGETATIVE . . . See autonomous.

VERTEBRATE . . . Any animal that has a back-bone.

For wholesale pricing on The HCG Weight Loss Cure Guide or on the following, simply contact us at www.PoundsAndInchesAway.com:

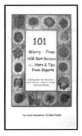

101-Worry Free Recipe Book

Recipe book features 101 recipes for main dishes, fruits, soups, drinks, and sauces which strictly adhere to Dr. Simeons' dietary guidelines and use ONLY ingredients approved on the original protocol. Copyright © 2008 by Linda Prinster (same author as HCG Weight Loss Cure Guide) and Leanne Mennemeier (successfully lost 46 pounds on the HCG Protocol). Both authors work extensively with HCG participants on a daily basis and continue to experience great success with the protocol.

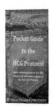

Pocket Guide to the HCG Protocol

Pocket guide provides a summarized version of the HCG Diet Protocol in purse/pocket size purely for convenience. This little book packs the basicHCG protocol information, and a nutrition chart of 1,000 items charting whether or not each item is allowed on each phase of the protocol. This small, summary book was created solely out of customer demand for a small resource to carry around. All information is extracted from The HCG Weight Loss Cure Guide.

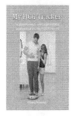

My HCG Tracker

Along with inspirational quotes to inspire you each day, *My HCG Tracker* helps you to easily track the foods you eat at each meal. This convenient and simple tracking allows you to see trends that may be causing your weight to stall or gain, an awareness which can ultimately increase your total weight loss.

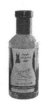

Pounds and Inches Away Dressing/Marinade

The **Pounds and Inches Away Vinaigrette** dressing is a approved for all phases of the HCG protocol including the VLCD (very low calorie diet days). This is great as a dressing for vegetables or a marinade for meat and is the only dressing we know of that is sweetened with stevia.

For more convenient, protocol-compliant products, go to www.HCGPerfectPortions.com.

Below are some samples of the products offered, which have been researched and tested for successful completion of the HCG Protocol. HCG Perfect Portions offers the ultimate in convenience and quality, yet strict adherence to Dr. Simeons' HCG Protocol.

 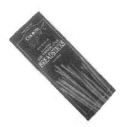 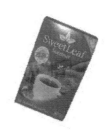 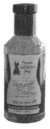

What other readers are saying:

The quality of these books are excellent - Where to get info is included - A++

HCG guide everything you need to get started - very detailed.

This is a must-have!

Good info - especially for new HCGers!!! Thank you!!!

This GUIDE is very helpful; better than the book by Kevin T. Thanks.

All-inclusive HCG info...couldn't ask for more...super easy...I'm on my way!!!

About the Author

My name is Linda Prinster. At the time of updating this book, I am a 45 year old mother of 8 children ranging from 23 years old to 3 year old. I have been married 25 years to the same man and, yes, all of the children are 'our' children.

I have struggled with weight my entire life. I am one of the strong, according to Dr. Simeons, as I have always known that while maintaining a specific, healthy weight was a struggle for my body, the struggle was not caused by what I improperly did or what I improperly ate. Although I would never be classified as obese on a weight chart, I did indeed have most or all of the 'signs and symptoms of obesity' Dr. Simeons so clearly defines.

I have dieted too many times to count over the years; some worked at least temporarily (NutriSystem worked until the formula was changed to not be such a high protein mix of nutrients; Atkins worked for weight loss, but the return of virtually any carbohydrates brought the slow return of the weight; diet pills made weight loss possible as long as I was taking the pills, but the side effects can be serious); some didn't work at all (Weight Watchers, 'cutting back and exercising more', walking, etc.).

We overweight people know that thin, metabolically blessed people simply don't believe this information, but that's o.k., there may come a day when they 'get it' – not that I would wish it upon anyone! By doctors, I have been described as extremely metabolically resistant. Doctors have explained that I have a body that knows how to survive like the cavemen – it will take what it can get and keep it just in case it needs it sometime in the future (thanks a lot!). But, I always searched and hoped for a better, more complete answer – enter HCG.

My qualifications in writing this guide include a PMP certification and significant consulting experience in management, research and documentation, and weight loss. Additionally, I owned and ran a 30 minute workout franchise for about 2 years before having my last 2 children within a short period. During this time, I ran Biggest Loser Contests and consulted many individuals – oh, how I wish I would have known about Dr. Simeons and HCG then. Finally, I personally experienced great results on Dr. Simeons Protocol (lost about 30 pounds and maintained the loss) and have consulted with hundreds of individuals on the protocol from start to finish. The overall results we see on a daily basis continue to impress us beyond our greatest expectations. To date, 99% of committed participants have had extraordinary success in both losing the weight, and even more importantly, most understand how to actually keep it off. I am able to eat far more now, and not gain weight, than I ever could in the past. As far as reshaping, HCG does it – I weigh 8-10 pounds more than I have in the past, but am comfortably in a size 8 for the FIRST TIME IN MY LIFE. HCG has performed better than I could have ever hoped for. For some, including me, this is 'the cure'.

I wish healthy weight, body, and mind to everyone undertaking this exciting method of weight loss. This guide, including Dr. Simeons HCG protocol, fully promotes a healthy, normal philosophy of life. The protocol promotes a drastic change in a quick time frame that has long term results. Most participants are quickly set free to enjoy a healthy life with normal eating and relatively little regard for unrealistic rules such as counting calories or anything else. Congratulations if you have chosen this path among the many paths – surely success will be yours and surely you will not be disappointed in your journey.

Made in the USA
Charleston, SC
19 August 2010